WHAT SHOULD I EAT?

COOKING FOR KITCHEN NEWBIES

First published in Australia in 2022 by Tedd Poulos
Text and photography copyright © Tedd Poulos 2022
The right of Tedd Poulos to be identified as the author of this
work has been asserted by him in accordance with the Copyright
Amendment (Moral Rights) Act 2000.

This work is copyrighted. Apart from any use as permitted under
the Copyright Act 1968, no part may be reproduced, copied, scanned,
stored in a retrieval system, recorded, or transmitted, in any form or
by any means, without the prior written permission of the publisher.

National Library of Australia Cataloguing-in-Publication data:
Poulos, Tedd, author.
What Should I Eat? : Cooking for Kitchen Newbies

 A catalogue record for this book is available from the National Library of Australia

ISBN: 978 0 6456665 0 2 (paperback)
ISBN: 978 0 6456665 2 6 (hardback)
ISBN: 978 0 6456665 1 9 (ebook)

Credits:
Food Director – Tedd Poulos
Photography & Styling – Tedd Poulos
Editors – Sasha Tropp and Paul Simmons
Project Designer – Liz Seymour
Proudly printed in Australia by Imagination Graphics Pty Ltd, Marrickville

WHAT SHOULD I EAT?

COOKING FOR KITCHEN NEWBIES

Tedd Poulos

ACKNOWLEDGEMENTS

To my family and friends who patiently and proudly support me to pursue new challenges like writing a book. I've been blessed that you have opened many doors that has allowed me to explore and accomplish amazing things that wouldn't have been possible otherwise. I'm incredibly grateful.

I have been coached and mentored by great people in sports and personal development. They have all shown me that finding your true potential is possible by reaching further than you think.

This book is dedicated to all of you.

CONTENTS

Introduction vii

About the author 1

How to use this book 2

Equipment & Utensils in Your Kitchen 4

Shopping for the Essentials 7

Keeping Your Non-stick Pans "Non-stick" 8

Sharpening Your Knife 11

Fresh Produce Explained 12

Tips, Tricks & Shortcuts for Your Lifestyle 22

Macronutrients & Calorie Calculator to Build Your Own Diet 25

Example of Daily Intake & Weekly Workouts 29

Consistency & Discipline 36

Summary 39

Breakfasts 43

Meals 61

Sides 93

Snacks 117

Smoothies & Juices 123

Macronutrient Breakdown 134

References 138

INTRODUCTION

You don't have to be an expert in the kitchen to take control of your meal preparation and get a handle on your nutrition. It will take less than three months to dial in your cooking and nutrition, at which point it becomes automatic for the rest of your life. It comes down to understanding what athletes and nutritionists already know. That is, knowing what to cook, how much to eat, and when to eat it. Simple, right?

I wasn't able to find a cookbook out there that teaches just the basics. I'm talking about the absolute essentials you need in your culinary arsenal. Sure, you have the Jamie Oliver Five-Ingredients-in-Five-Minutes type of books, but these are not the basic recipes that I'm talking about. I needed meals that were easy to remember and would become second nature. With an athletic background, I needed meals that provided the fuel and recovery to sustain my level of activity.

Now I have them in this book. My meals work with my weekly shopping list, they fuel my fitness routine, and I'm never worried about what to cook next. They give me enough variety every week that I don't feel the need to deviate from the foods that I can cook, and I actually even impress people from time to time. It's much smarter and easier on your wallet when your fridge and pantry are stocked. When you know what to do with the food you buy, you can really take control of your health and well-being.

As a single guy with an active lifestyle and a big appetite, the basics are fast and keep me full. For a long time, food was just fuel to me, so microwaved rice and roasted chicken was usually on the menu. Food preparation throughout the week was normal and still is. The difference now is that I embraced learning to cook and can make foods that are just as healthy and that I actually enjoy!

These days, I cook things like ocean trout with chilli, lime, and ginger; angel hair pasta with homemade tomato sauce; and tabouli. Other days I make huge chicken wraps with raspberries and cashews and smoothies to go. My three goals in cooking are speed, maximum nutritional intake, and enjoyable to eat. Being efficient around the kitchen has taken away the chore of meal preparation. Cooking several dinners and lunches at one time is just automatic.

> This book is aimed at educating those who don't really know how to cook. It will break down what equipment is useful to own, what are good fresh produce options to buy, and how to take the guesswork out of what to cook next.

I used to be one of these people. I actually thought cooking many different meals required too many ingredients and I just wasn't equipped to handle it. It was overwhelming, so I just continued to struggle.

I wrote this book to be a personal guide to cooking basics and to get you started with your own development as a home cook. I'm not promising a revolutionary cookbook with ingredients that are new and innovative. Quite the opposite. These are the bare-bones tools needed to cook several breakfasts, lunches, and dinners for your household. My passions are health and fitness, so you will find that this book is your starter's guide to nutrition and weight management too. Now that I've introduced a greater diversity of superfoods into my meal plans, my physique and athletic performance has soared to another level. More importantly, my overall health and energy has noticeably improved! That's what I want for you.

I hope you enjoy this book and take something away from it.

Tedd Poulos

NOTE: I don't often eat foods with creams, sauces, butter, and gravy or that are deep fried. There's too much sugar and fat in those things and I just don't want that. I actually prefer fresh produce and meals with clean calories that taste amazing and make me feel better. My recipes do not always contain traditional ingredients, and I substitute certain ingredients for things that I buy weekly. Sure, I'll make an exception when I know I want to try a meal that requires something out of the ordinary, and I'll remember to buy the specific ingredients for it that week. But typically, keeping it simple and consistent keeps me on track. This is not a strict diet book, and you should definitely substitute ingredients if they cause you problems.

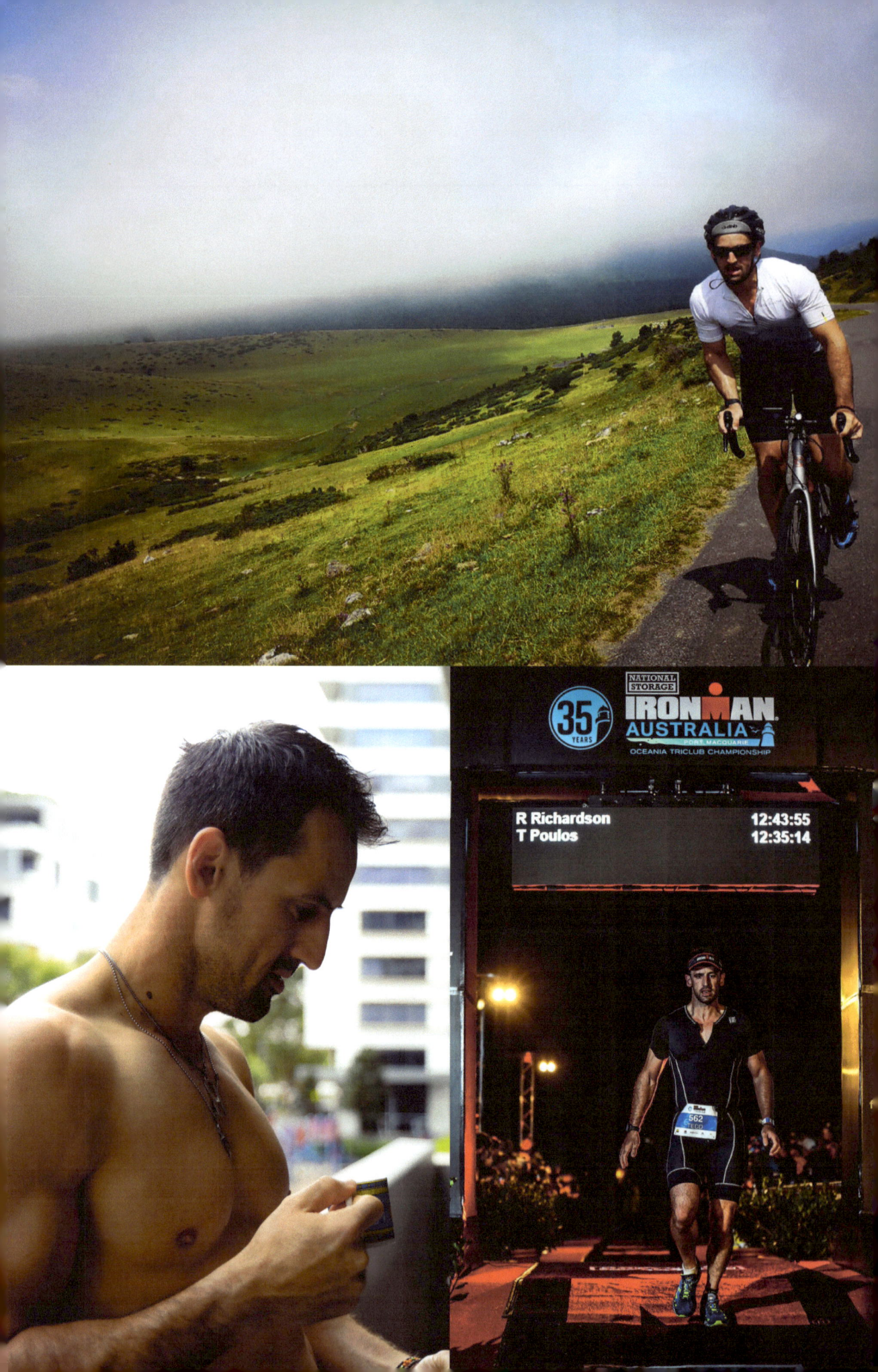

ABOUT THE AUTHOR

I don't think my adult life has changed too much from my childhood. My hobbies and passions are just more expensive now. I was a busy kid who focused on school and sports. I was lucky to have natural talent in both, but I spent all my time studying or training. A little bit of success at school encouraged me to keep chasing new goals. This confidence spilt over into my sports and my enjoyment of sports stuck with me year after year.

Now, in 2022, I'm 38 years old. I find myself having a career in construction that is incredibly enjoyable. My passions are in health and fitness more than ever. I love the process of learning new skills, and I've bounced from one sporting project to another.

The single most significant turning point, or really springboard moment, was competing in bodybuilding in 2011. An opportunity came to me to have a personal coach who taught me about nutrition and eating for 14 weeks. It was only then that I actually learnt about macro nutritional breakdowns, calories, sugar, weight loss, and muscle gain. It was an experience like nothing else to step on stage incredibly lean when my stomach was as tight as the skin on the back of your hand!

I definitely developed cooking and eating habits that I still adhere to today. Over those three months of preparation, I learnt about portion control, calorie intake, and weight management. I learnt that the ideal meal plan is the one that you can sustain year after year. For overall health, food needs to be nutritious and taste great.

So I set out to write a cookbook for myself. I actually wanted to be good at making the foods I wanted to eat, rather than be limited to a diet of only what I could cook. I enjoyed the process of learning my way around the kitchen and then took on the challenge of documenting everything. A creative project away from my routine of training and work was a welcome change.

I knew from the beginning that this cookbook could take beginners from nowhere to somewhere and fast track those who would otherwise take 10 years or more to learn like I did.

HOW TO USE THIS BOOK

The purpose of this book is not to show off ground-breaking recipes, but to be used as a one-stop shop for kitchen newbies to learn to cook staple meals using a typical weekly shopping list. It takes the guess work out of cooking. I touch on basic nutritional and health information to make sense of it all and answer why to even eat these foods at all! My thought is that if you understand why your health depends on eating a variety of fresh produce then you will give more priority to cooking and remember several homemade options for breakfast, lunch, dinner, and snacks in between.

Secondly, it describes exactly how to build your own meal plan. Meal portion sizes are not discussed very often in cooking, but it really goes hand in hand with the food you eat when you are mindful of your weight. I describe how to calculate your required daily calorie intake and what macronutrients mean. All of the recipes have a macronutrient breakdown and calorie value which describes my portion sizes; you should adjust the grams per serving to suit yourself.

It's difficult for authors to publish recipes with serving sizes because every person's needs are different. However, I do include them on this occasion as an example for you. My portion sizes are on the high side of the calorie requirement for most people since I exercise regularly. There are a few things you should do if you want to model your meal plan off my recipes:

1. Calculate your own daily calorie requirement. See page 26.
2. Increase the number of servings in the recipes which reduces the calories per serving
3. Adjust the recipes to reduce the high-calorie ingredients. See the summary table on page 136.

Every cookbook I've browsed includes fantastic recipes that are restaurant-quality. The problem for us beginners is that these meals require a long list of ingredients. That includes ingredients I don't buy, ingredients I've never heard of, and ingredients that I just don't like. So how will I ever learn and remember to make them? This book works with a consistent shopping list that becomes easy to remember over time. There will be the odd ingredient to buy from time to time when you plan your weekly meals and others that can be stored for a while, like flour and breadcrumbs. I encourage you to learn from my list and then modify it as your own.

I live a healthy lifestyle, but chicken and rice become boring very quickly. I've learnt that food can be completely healthy and still packed with flavour. I started to design this book for young singles and those who don't really know how to cook. Then I figured people who needed guidance for weight management could take a lot from it too. Weight management is for everyone, and it's not about going on a diet. It's about lifestyle and consistency over time. In fact, consistency and discipline are my buzz words. We're going back to basics and

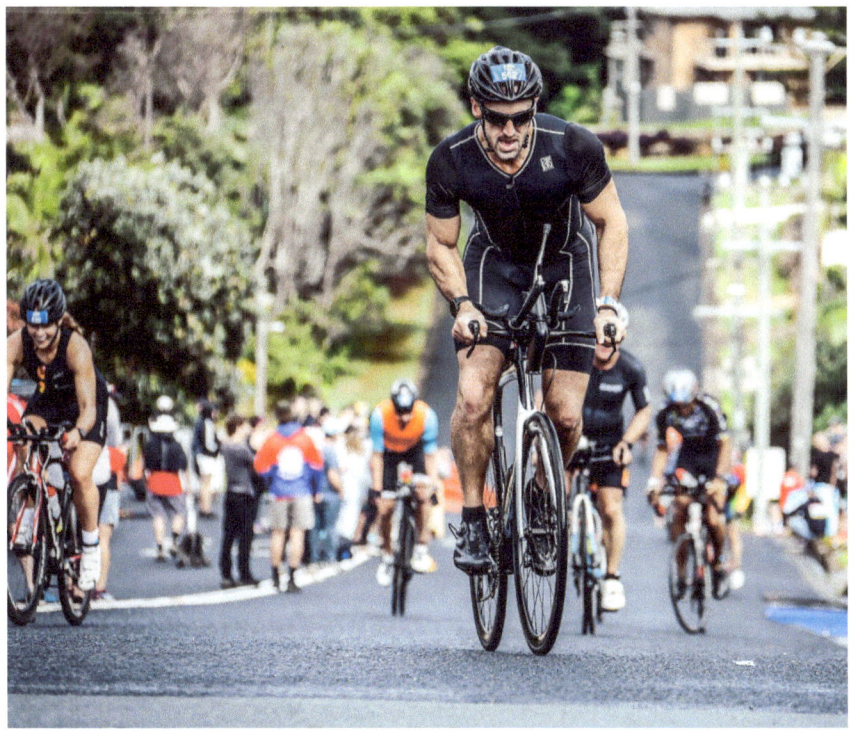

we're going to do them well! We will keep our lives simple by making shopping and cooking easy, and you can try different combinations of protein and carbohydrate sources when building your own meals. I'm going to show you that there's nothing wrong with learning the basics because it's going to get you on track. Cooking is simple when you know how. I've mostly put away typical cookbooks and written my own because it's what I know I can stick to seven days a week. And it's not a big deal when you do eat out on the weekend when you want to socialise with friends.

Don't be put off by the straight forward recipe titles. There's plenty of variety and combinations in here to keep your meals interesting and keep you on a clean path. The best advice is to follow the rule of thirds and to fill your plate with ⅓ protein, ⅓ carbohydrates, ⅓ vegetables, along with some healthy fats. Any combination will work. What's important is your portion size. So if you like potatoes with your steak, then do that. If you like rice instead, then that's okay too. It's the same thing. Just remember your portion size!

What Should I Eat? is for anyone who hates that feeling of deciding what to make for dinner. It takes out the guesswork when you can primarily stick to the same shopping list each week and simply build your meals within a structure.

EQUIPMENT & UTENSILS IN YOUR KITCHEN

Success in the kitchen will come, and a big advantage is having all of the necessary tools at your fingertips. This is a quick list of everything you will need.

NON-STICK OVEN TRAYS × 2

Two large oven trays (approximately 44cm × 32cm / 7.75L) will be used for all of your baking. Meals you can bake means you can cook in bulk without standing over your stove for hours. Using baking paper to line the trays means cleaning is as easy as throwing the paper away.

NON-STICK FRYING PAN × 1 LARGE

One large pan (approximately 32cm in diameter) will be your go-to for all of your stove cooking. A large pan allows you to cook in bulk as well as make smaller meals for one. This pan should be well looked after and used correctly so that it lasts for years. (Read more on that in chapter 5 - Keeping Your Non-Stick Pans "Non-Stick".)

NON-STICK SAUCEPAN × 1 SMALL

It took me a while to come around to a small saucepan (approximately 18cm / 2.5L), but I like it for preparing sauces and mixing in pasta. Saucepans are deeper than a frying pan but shallower than a pot. They're good for heating and cooking liquids on a stovetop because the high sides stop liquids from spilling and their smaller size with a single handle is easy to handle. Saucepans are good for bringing liquids to a boil much more quickly than large pots.

NON-STICK POT × 1 LARGE

You need one large pot with a steamer basket (approximately 26cm / 11L) for boiling water to cook large quantities of rice, pasta, vegetables and potatoes when cooking for multiple meals. Pots have deep sides and two handles. Pots can hold larger volumes of liquids and food than pans and saucepans and they suit meals that require longer cooking times. While pots and saucepans are interchangeable, pots aren't typically used for cooking sauces because they don't heat small quantities as well and therefore extend the cooking time.

ELECTRIC OR MICROWAVE RICE COOKER

Using a rice cooker is the most time-effective way to cook rice and is much easier to clean than a pot. You can really set and forget with a rice cooker, allowing you to continue preparing other parts of your meal without checking on it. One advantage of a rice cooker is that they keep your rice warm for hours if you put it on early.

GLOBAL KNIFE (& WHETSTONE FOR SHARPENING) × 1

A good-quality knife (I use a Global Classic G-2 20cm chef's knife) is a pleasure to use. Cutting your food with a sharp knife is effortless and safest to use. It's frustrating to use a knife that just doesn't do the job. There's a noticeable difference in using a quality knife over a cheap knife. If you need to justify spending money on it and a whetstone for sharpening, consider that you will use it on a daily basis for years to come. It's worth the money.

SLAP CHOP (HAND OPERATED DICER)

A slap-chop is a TV shopping product which is an absolute gem! Firstly, it works and does exactly what the TV commercial says. It is small and portable and dices your food in seconds by pressing down on the spring-loaded handle. It is extremely useful for finely chopping garlic, mushrooms, herbs, and chilli. The best part is that it is easy to clean. Slap-chops take out the effort and time spent doing this type of preparation with a knife.

900W NUTRIBULLET BLENDER

A NutriBullet blender or similar is another must-have in the kitchen. I use mine daily for shakes and juices and then other times for meal preparation. The size of the cup suits the size of tall protein shakers so I can make a smoothie and transfer to a shaker cup when I'm in a rush out the door.

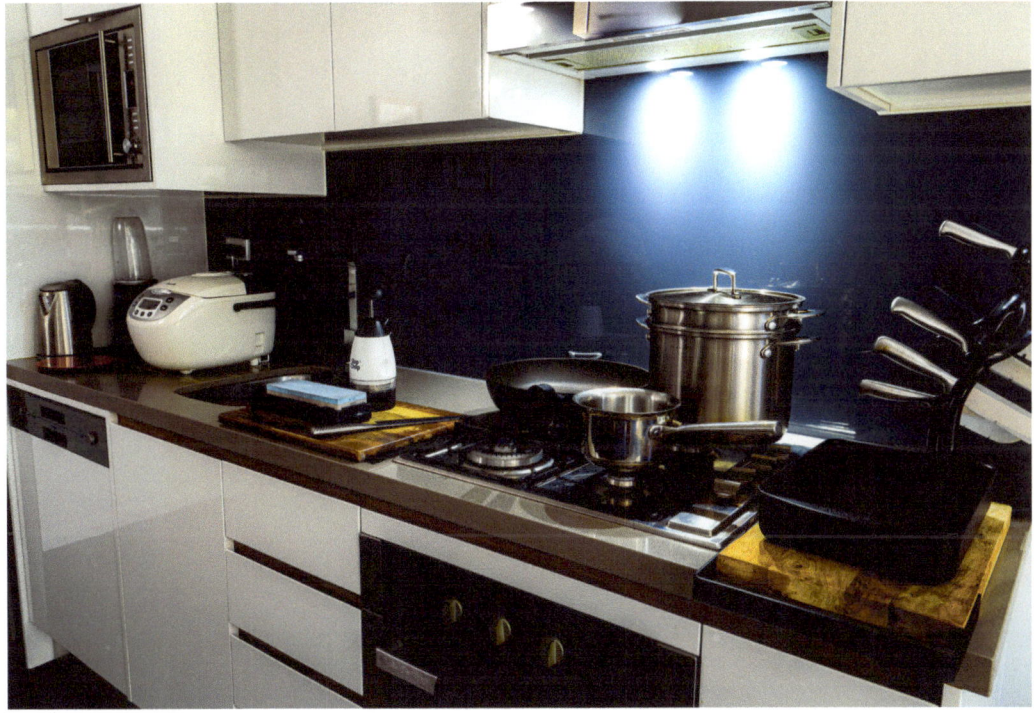

MORTAR & PESTLE

This is a new addition in my kitchen. I like using it to crush and mix herbs and spices for barbeque rubs and chimichurri sauces.

KITCHEN SCALES

Kitchen scales are a must when you're starting to learn about calories and portion sizes. It's one thing to read "200g chicken breast" in a recipe, but what does that really look like? Most recipes are measured in cup and spoon sizes, but scales are obviously useful for protein sizes which are typically described in grams.

RANGE OF KITCHEN UTENSILS AND APPLIANCES

It's no surprise that a range of utensils will come in handy at different times. Generally, you should have on hand a potato peeler, measuring cups, measuring spoons, kitchen scissors, plastic spatulas, plastic tongs, a can opener, a grater, wooden spoons, and clips for sealing packs. Do I need to mention a kettle and toaster too?

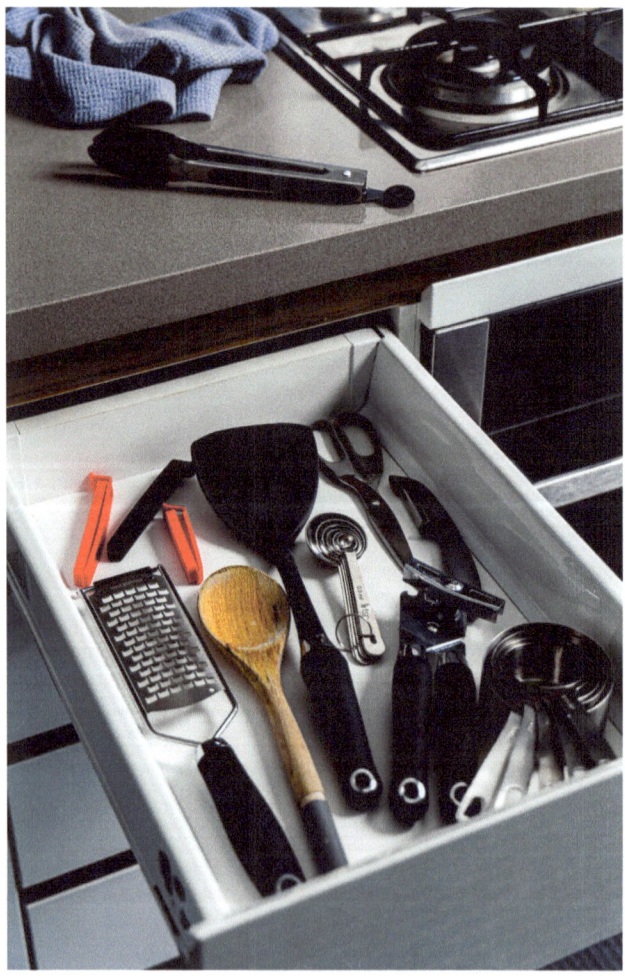

SHOPPING FOR THE ESSENTIALS

Below is a full list of ingredients in this book and regular staples in my fridge and pantry. I keep it relatively simple and shop for the same things each week. Writing your shopping list is a great idea to start out; once you see a list of ingredients, you'll realise how many combinations there are for meals. Shopping then becomes automatic after time. The best advice I can give you if you want to build your own shopping list is that you need to eat what you like. The foods that I consistently go to are mostly low in calorie density and high in nutrient value, and I thoroughly enjoy eating everything listed here. It's a major reason why I'm able to maintain my athletic physique and overall health.

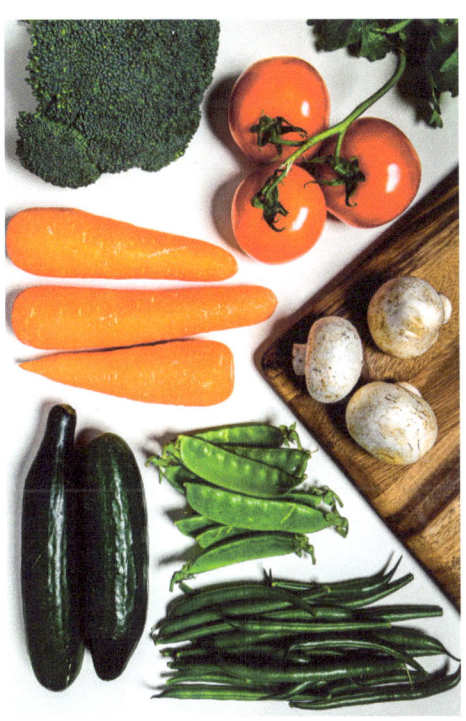

PROTEIN
Beef
Pork
Seafood
Chicken
Turkey
Kangaroo
Eggs
Yogurt
Protein powder

CARBOHYDRATES
Oats
Rice
Couscous
Potato
Sweet potato
Pasta
Bread
Noodles

FATS
Olive oil
Coconut oil
Peanut oil
Peanut butter
Avocado
Almonds, cashews & macadamia nuts

FRUIT
Apples
Kiwi
Oranges
Lemons
Limes
Bananas
Passionfruit
Blueberries
Raspberries
Strawberries
Pineapple
Watermelon
Frozen mixed berries

FRESH HERBS
Parsley
Basil
Oregano
Mint
Dill
Thyme
Rosemary

VEGETABLES
Celery
Ginger
Garlic
Mushrooms
Leafy greens
Tomatoes
Cucumber
Broccoli
Corn
Beans
Snow peas
Carrot
Shallots
Chilli
Olives
Capsicum
Beetroot

SPICES
Cinnamon
Paprika
Chilli flakes

OTHER STAPLES
Honey
Tea & coffee
Milk
Tuna cans
Rice packs
Salt & pepper
Flour
Breadcrumbs
Bicarb soda
Greens superfood powder
Psyllium husk
Flaxseed powder
Cocoa powder
Dark chocolate, 70%
Muesli
Chia seeds
Passata
Crushed tomatoes
Sesame oil
Soy sauce
Bulgar
Vanilla extract
Feta cheese
Chicken stock

KEEPING YOUR NON-STICK PANS "NON-STICK"

Preventing food from sticking to your pan depends on how you "season" or treat your pans, cooking temperature, and general cleaning rules. You have the choice of non-stick pans, stainless steel, and cast-iron.

NON-STICK PANS

Non-stick pans have a non-stick coating. There are several types to consider. Ceramic-coated pans do not leach chemicals into food, making them the safest for home use on low to medium heat. They retain heat well and distribute it evenly.

The most common non-stick surface is polytetrafluroethylene (PTFE), commonly referred to as Teflon. Like ceramic coatings, it's suited to low to medium heat but sensitive to scratches and damage from high heat. There has been some controversy regarding whether Teflon pans may be toxic if exposed to prolonged high heat. However, PTFE coatings manufactured after 2013 do not contain PFOA (perfluorooctanoic acid), making them a safe choice nowadays. Check this before buying a PTFE pan.

Manufacturers and experts say no matter how much you baby your non-stick pans, their life expectancy is three to five years. They lack durability and are prone to scratches. My pan is going on five years now and is starting to show some wear.

Rules for general use

Only use low to medium cooking temperatures. High temperatures ruin the non-stick coating.

Do not use spray cooking oils. It actually has the opposite effect of what you would think. It leaves a film that makes the pan less slick. It's okay to use cooking oils like olive oil to enhance the non-stick quality.

Use plastic or wooden utensils and absolutely no metal. Anything sharp or rough on your pan will scratch the ceramic coating.

Rules for cleaning

Do not put your pan in the dishwasher. It slowly wears the ceramic coating.

Use warm, soapy water and a soft sponge. Do not use an abrasive sponge which will remove the ceramic non-stick coating.

Wash when your pan is cool.

STAINLESS STEEL PANS

Stainless steel pans are the pan of choice for chefs. They are more durable than non-stick pans and last a lifetime, especially when seasoned and used correctly. And, of course, they are non-stick.

Rules for seasoning the pan

Heat the pan to a high temperature. As it's heating, add coconut oil which has a high smoking point, meaning it won't burn away. Move the pan to allow the oil to cover the bottom and sides. When the oil starts smoking, take it off the heat and remove the excess oil with paper towel. Seasoning your pan this way will keep it non-stick for months to come.

Rules for general use

Stainless steel pans are temperature sensitive like non-stick pans. Too low, and food will stick; too high, and it will stick and burn.

Use the mercury test to find the right cooking temperature. Heat the pan to medium heat. Use two to three drops of water. If the temperature is too low, the water will evaporate. If the temperature is too high, the water will splatter inside the pan. The drops of water will bead in the pan when the temperature is right.

Only use low to medium cooking temperatures. It's okay to use cooking oils like olive oil.

Any utensils are okay to use since there isn't an applied non-stick coating.

Rules for cleaning

Stainless steel pans are dishwasher-safe. Hand-washing is still the ideal option.

When there's minimum grime, using warm and soapy water with a sponge is sufficient.

Again, note that cooking temperatures that are too high will cause food to stick and burn. Using abrasive sponges when needed is okay. They will leave fine scratch marks, but it has no effect on the longevity of your pan.

When your pan is really dirty, a cheap trick is to use baking soda as an abrasive cleaner. Pour a generous mound in the centre of the pan on medium heat. Pour water around the mound and watch it come to boil. The baking soda will start to react and evaporate around the pan, breaking down all the food bits and making it much easier to scrub clean.

CAST-IRON PANS

Cast-iron pans like most barbeque plates are another option. The advantage of using a cast-iron pan is that you can cook things like steaks at higher temperatures. They last a lifetime and are non-stick when seasoned correctly. The disadvantage of these pans is that they do require a little more care in seasoning and cleaning and take longer to heat up.

Rules for seasoning the pan

Again, seasoning your pan is crucial. Flaxseed oil is the best to use for seasoning; canola oil is cheaper and okay to use. While heating the pan on the stove, wipe the oil over all sides, not just the cooking surface. Cast-iron pans are made of a single piece of iron, so the whole outside of the pan and handle can be seasoned also.

Preheat your oven to its highest temperature or at least 400'°C. Place the pan upside down (this prevents the oil from pooling) in the oven for an hour. The oil absorbs into the pores of the cast-iron and will give the pan a glass-like non-stick surface.

Rules for general use

Cast-iron pans take time to heat. One mistake you might make is trying to cook the food when the pan isn't hot enough. Let your pan heat first, then apply cooking oil and throw in your ingredients.

A tip for cooking protein like chicken or steaks is not to move the meat around the pan too soon. The meat will stick to the pan early on. Let it cook and it will release from the pan once it develops a crusty layer.

Cast-iron cookware is so durable that it's fine to use with metal utensils. Silicon spatulas are fine to use as well; however, stainless steel utensils are preferable for their durability and versatility.

Another advantage of cast iron pans is that you can start cooking your meal on the stove and then finish it in the oven.

Rules for cleaning

Wash when the pan is warm. You can use abrasive sponges and the baking soda trick described above to loosen food stuck in the pan. Hot, soapy water is generally okay to use to clean these pans.

The most important thing to remember is that water causes cast-iron pans to rust, so ensure they are properly dried before storing. You can even put them in the oven again to dry. Protect your pan in between uses by applying a layer of oil and heating it on the stove until the oil starts to smoke.

OVEN TRAYS

Baking paper is your friend! We can keep this section short and say that you should use and clean as above, but the advantage with the oven is that you can use baking paper to line your trays. They stay clean every single time. Use and throw away the paper. I rarely need to wipe up anything more than excess seasoning and oil from my trays.

SHARPENING YOUR KNIFE

Invest in at least one quality knife. You are preparing food daily so it's worth every dollar. I was gifted a Global Knife Global Classic G-2 20cm chef's knife and it's my "cuts everything" knife. Slicing a tomato with ease is the ultimate test for a knife, and you'll agree that these are the best.

Even these quality knives dull over time and require maintenance in the form of sharpening. So the second thing I encourage you to invest in is a whetstone. I use my whetstone approximately every one to two months and it takes just a small number of passes to keep the blade razor-sharp.

Whetstones are described by grit. Find one that is double-sided, something like 1,000/5,000 grit. The higher the number, the finer the sharpening. For example, if you need to completely restore a dull blade, you should use the rougher 1,000 grit stone first and then fine-tune the sharpening with the finer 5,000 grit stone.

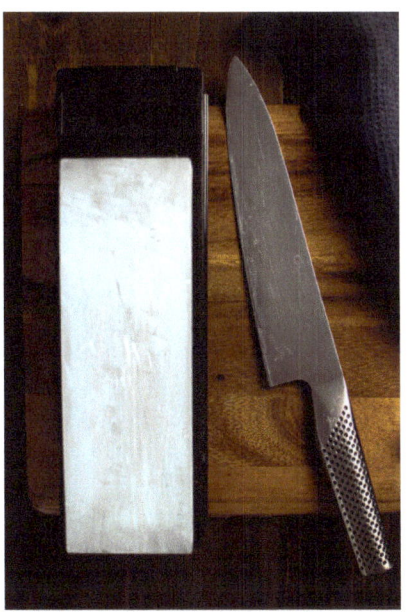

Whetstones must be kept wet when using. The mud on top of the stone is what sharpens the knife. Before using the stone, submerge it in water in your sink. Give it a few minutes, until you no longer see any air bubbles coming out of the stone.

Keep the stone on top of a tea towel on your chopping board. Raise it off the bench on the whetstone case or the edge of a chopping board to give your hand more clearance when you start sharpening.

A few things to remember:
1. Keep the blade at the same angle during each pass. This goes for both sides of the blade.
2. Sharpen the first side by keeping the blade at a 45-degree angle to the whetstone and apply pressure while moving the knife with your whole arm, from your elbow and shoulder.
3. Focus on long strokes to sharpen the whole length of the blade.
4. Apply pressure to sharpen in both directions away from and towards your body.
5. Keep the stone wet by dripping water onto it during sharpening.
6. I like to sharpen the reverse side by keeping it at a 90-degree angle to the stone. In theory, this creates the cutting teeth in the knife.
7. Continue alternating equally for 5 to 10 minutes on each side.
8. Watch YouTube to see this technique and others in action. YouTube "sharpening with a whetstone" for excellent demonstrations.

FRESH PRODUCE EXPLAINED

Macronutrients are the primary nutrition categories that your diet is built around. Your metabolism is like an engine that needs fuel to keep it ticking. I subscribe to a balanced approach and focus on taking in a portion of protein, carbohydrates, and fat in each meal. Being as active as I am, my meals are every two to three hours.

Put simply, I want protein for muscle repair, carbohydrates for energy, fruit and vegetables for their anti-inflammatory and antioxidant qualities to boost strong immunity to fight disease, and healthy fats for their anti-aging and disease-fighting qualities. All these foods play a role in overall health and I need all of these things to cater to my active lifestyle. Even without an active lifestyle, you can eat yourself healthy with each of these types of foods. Modifying your portion sizes and calories to suit your activity level is what's important.

PROTEINS

Don't get caught up with worrying about which protein source is the best. They are all clean options and basically have the same amount of protein. It's more important to focus on giving your body variety. Protein is important to our immune system, to rebuilding muscle, and even to controlling hunger. The rule of thumb is 1.7g of protein per kilogram of body weight each day.

Chicken, 200g = 45g protein
Pork, 200g = 48g protein
Salmon, 200g = 41g protein
Beef, 200g = 40g protein
Turkey, 200g = 43g protein
Kangaroo, 200g = 40g protein
Yogurt, 3 tbs (160g) = 14g protein
Protein powder, 30g scoop = 22g protein

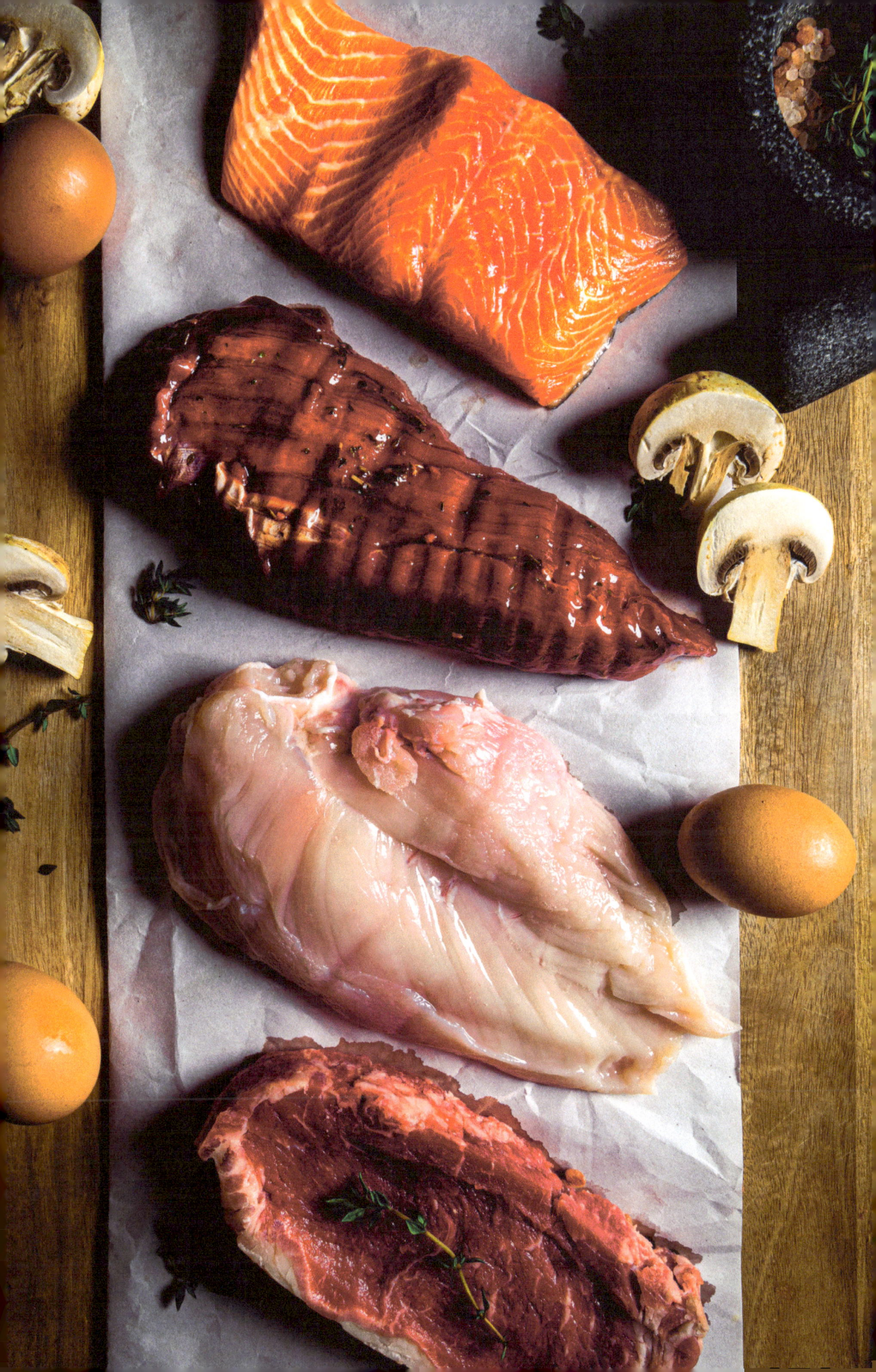

CARBOHYDRATES

Carbohydrates need to be included in your meal plan. For me, I need them to a large degree for long term success in athletic performance and physique goals. They come in the form of simple sugars, starches, and fibrous carbohydrates.

One reason why carbohydrates have a bad reputation for weight gain is that we tend to overeat them. They taste good and don't always satisfy our hunger. Before we know it, we blow out our portion size and eat too many calories.

Sugary carbs are the ones to avoid. They are hidden in processed foods like frozen dinners, fruit drinks, pasta sauce, and sweets. Anything in a packet or bottle really. The fructose component of sugar is undetected by the body and doesn't trigger our appetite control function, meaning we can eat them without feeling full.

Fibrous carbohydrates include all the vegetables that have a stabilising effect on your appetite and leave you feeling full. Starchy carbohydrates include rice, pasta, oats, and potatoes which are digested slowly. These carbohydrates are important for feeling energetic and healthy and for maintaining your goal weight. They do come with risks, as we can overeat them, but you just need to be aware of how much you eat.

Carbohydrates shouldn't be avoided. I almost never leave carbohydrates out of a meal. Your brain alone takes a significant amount of energy to function. A strong workout or long run depends on having fuel in the tank which carbs deliver. Don't over complicate things by associating carbohydrates with weight gain. Training with intensity makes fat loss possible, not training with an empty gas tank. Calorie control should be your focus and your portion sizes should be in line with your level of exercise and goals.

Oats, 1 cup = 70g carbohydrates
Rice, 1 cup = 58g carbohydrates
Potato, 1 cup = 22g carbohydrates
Sweet potato, 1 cup = 34g carbohydrates
Pasta, 1 cup = 79g carbohydrates
Sourdough bread, 2 slices = 24g carbohydrates

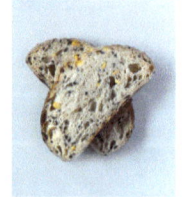
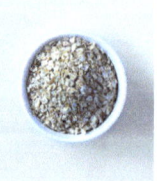
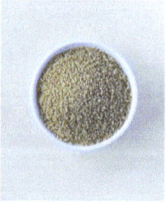
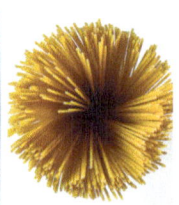
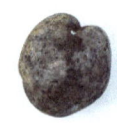
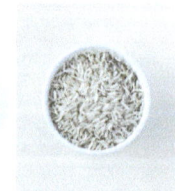

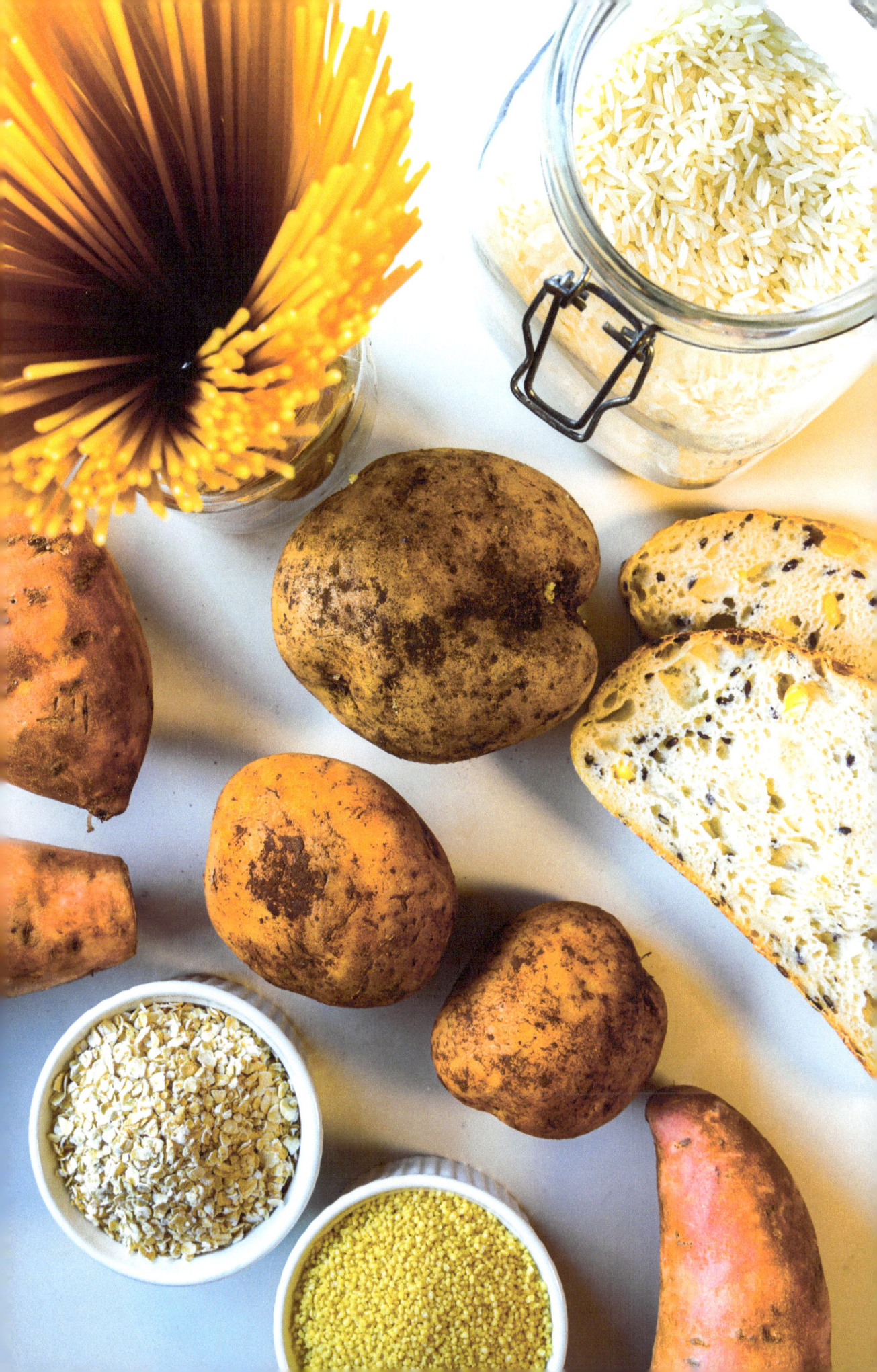

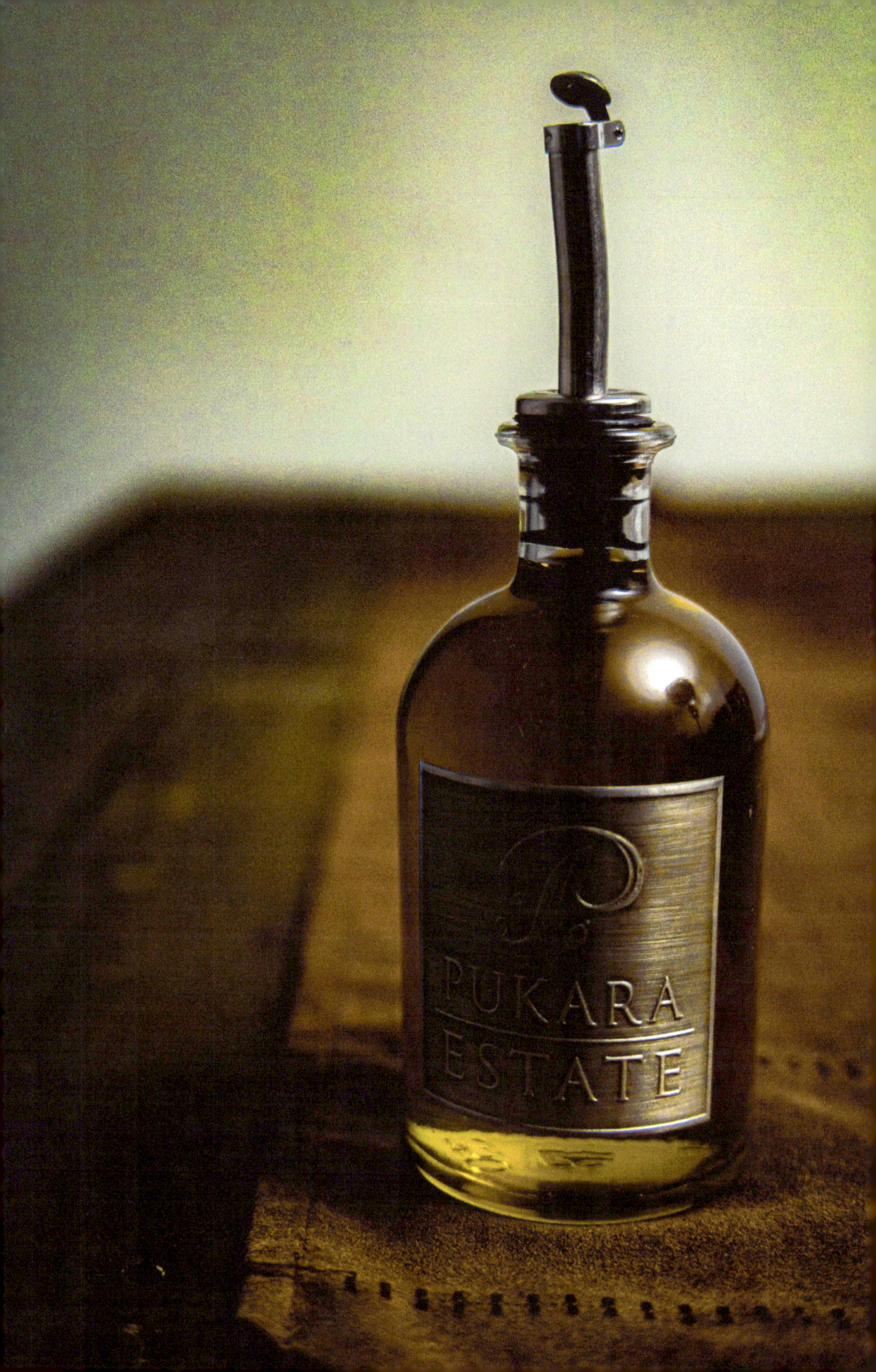

FATS

Incorporating healthy fats like olive oil, peanut butter, salmon, avocado, and nuts into your diet will have you feeling full and energetic. I used to think I could get leaner by avoiding these fats, but I only felt lethargic and tired. Now that I follow a balanced meal plan that includes 25% fats, I'm still lean and far more alert and energetic.

Look at studies for the past thirty years about the health benefits of different fats. Healthy fats like avocados, coconut oil, and olive oil are essential antioxidants for fighting disease and controlling aging in the skin, resulting in a youthful complexion. It's proven that we live longer and live healthier when we consume healthy fats.

Olive oil protects the body from the inflammatory effects of toxins which damage our cells. Use olive oil to dress salads and only cook with it on a low to moderate heat. When oils start to burn at too high of a temperature, they degrade and produce smoke. The fat molecules break apart and turn into various harmful compounds and some flavour can be lost. Thankfully olive oil is suited to most cooking and is quite resistant to heat. Furthermore, it's one of the healthiest oils.

Peanut oil is ideal for stir-fries and cooking at higher temperatures. It has a higher smoking point than olive oil which means it will not burn and turn to smoke on higher heat. Peanut oil also doesn't interfere with the flavour of the food.

Olive oil, 1 tbs = 14g fat
Peanut oil, 1 tbs = 14g fat
Peanut butter, 1 tbs = 10g fat
Avocado, medium (160g) = 34g fat
Cashew nuts, 30g = 15g fat

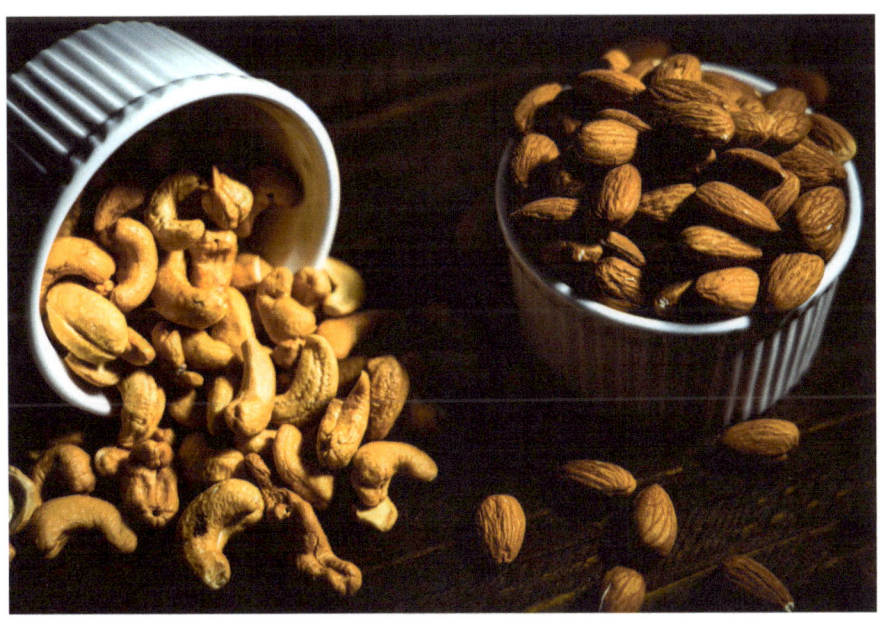

FRUIT / VEGETABLES / HERBS & SPICES

Remember that fruit, vegetables, herbs, and spices are all superfoods. Each of them contains healing powers for your body, satisfy cravings in between meals, and help you manage stress. They are nature's way to detox your skin and help us all age gracefully. It's not a secret that they are one key component to your overall health so make a specific effort to include these foods into your day. It's just not enough to just eat them here or there.

The Australian Heart Foundation recommends that we consume two servings of fruit and five servings of vegetables per day. A serving of fruit is simply a piece of fruit or a fruit juice. A serving of vegetables is ½ cup of cooked vegetables, 1 cup of raw or salad vegetables, or half of a potato. Eating more fruit is easy if you just add it to your meals like I describe in my recipes. The rule of thirds, described in chapter 8 - Tips, Tricks & Shortcuts for Your Lifestyle, is the best rule to follow to ensure that vegetables always find their way onto your plate. Drinking a vegetable juice like my Green Juice (see page 131) is the easiest way to get your daily dose of vegetables.

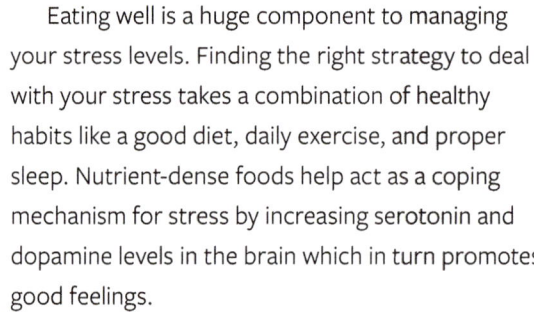

Eating well is a huge component to managing your stress levels. Finding the right strategy to deal with your stress takes a combination of healthy habits like a good diet, daily exercise, and proper sleep. Nutrient-dense foods help act as a coping mechanism for stress by increasing serotonin and dopamine levels in the brain which in turn promotes good feelings.

I recommend buying fresh herbs, fruits, and vegetables from your greengrocer. You do pay a little more than at the supermarket, but the quality is far better and the food will last longer. The same goes for meat and fish; buy them at your local butcher and seafood shop. The supermarket will cover the rest.

My approach to these foods is to take a little in with each meal. Smoothies are handy because you can blend so many superfoods into one quick and delicious drink to get your daily dose on the run.

Medical Medium: Life-Changing Foods by Anthony William is an excellent book about the biochemistry that the Holy Four (fruit / vegetables / herbs / spices) create within your body. It goes into detail about the healing power of these foods and how they bring emotional and spiritual benefits.

Tips for storing:
- Refrigerate fresh parsley, basil, and mint wrapped in paper towels in airtight containers.
- Refrigerate vegetables like tomatoes, cucumbers, and carrots in plastic bags.
- Fruits can be stored at room temperature out of direct sunlight. Having said that, berries and cut fruit like watermelon and pineapple should be refrigerated.

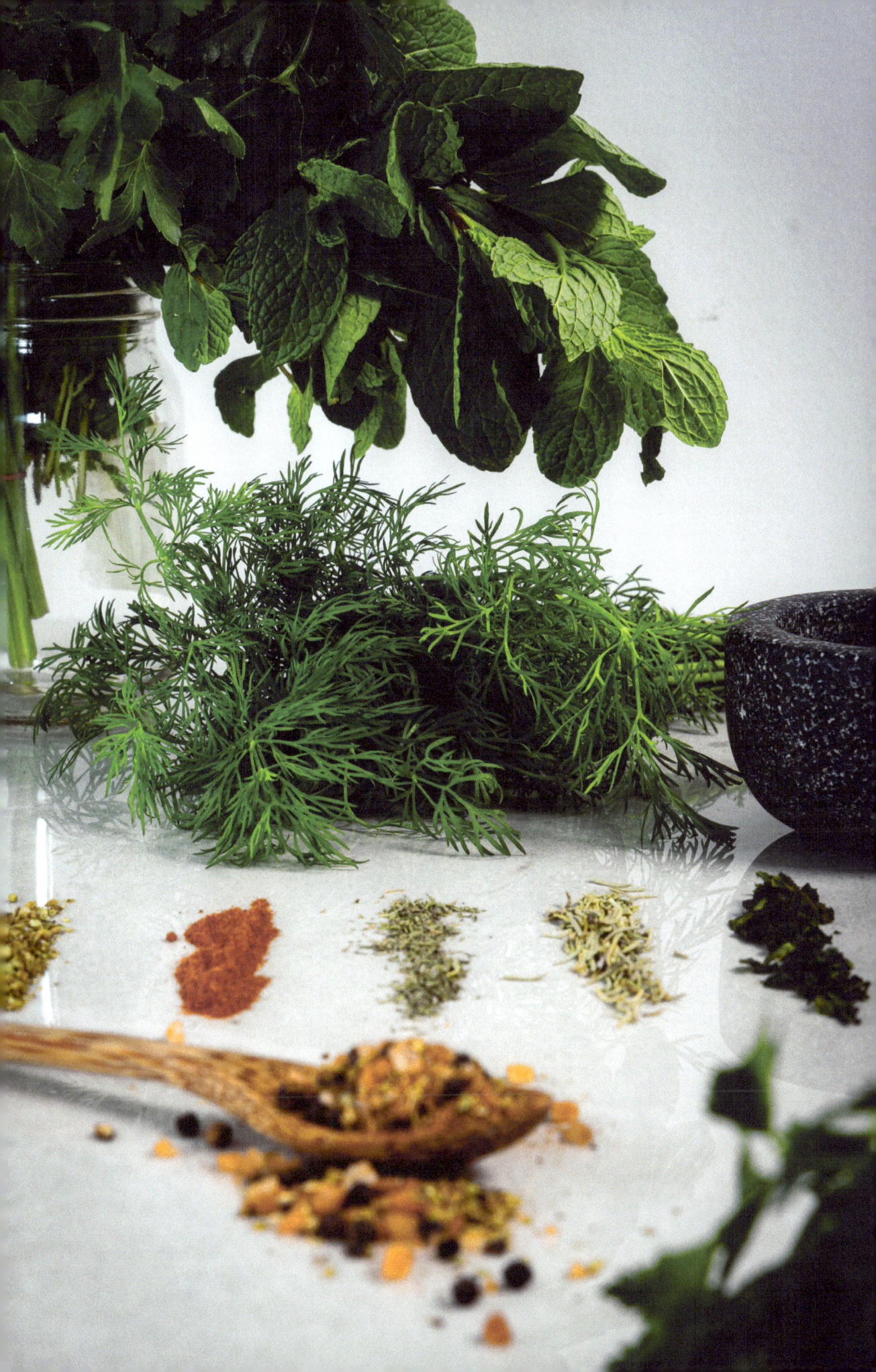

ANTI-INFLAMMATORY–RICH FOODS

Anti-inflammatory–rich foods include fresh produce like vegetables and fruit, fatty fish like salmon, and foods containing omega-3, such as olive oil, nuts, grains, seeds, and avocados. The term "anti-inflammatory" simply refers to the body's immune response against infection and injury. The more you fuel your body with these foods, the better your body's immunity will be to fight off disease, reduce the impact of injuries, and maintain a healthy weight. Reducing inflammation builds our cells and improves our organs' and skin's structure. All of these benefits are major contributors in controlling the speed of aging.

Examples of anti-inflammatory foods in this book include:

Vegetables & Fruit	Healthy Fats	Herbs
Broccoli	Chia seeds	Ginger
Potatoes	Almonds	Cinnamon
Green leafy vegetables like spinach	Avocado	Garlic
Strawberries	Salmon	Chilli
Blueberries	Ocean trout	
Raspberries	Olive oil	

ANTIOXIDANT-RICH FOODS

Antioxidants go hand in hand with anti-inflammatories; they act before inflammation even kicks in. Antioxidants protect our tissues from damage. By preventing infection in the first place, an anti-inflammatory response is not needed.

As a rule of thumb, foods high in antioxidants and anti-inflammatory properties are colourful fresh fruit and vegetables as well as those healthy fats previously mentioned. By cutting out refined sugar and processed (packaged) foods, you are more likely to pick foods that land in the antioxidant/anti-inflammatory category. They nourish our muscles, bones, hair, and skin. They keep our gut firing to better absorb the nutrients that our cells need to function. High-nutrient and antioxidant foods are important for overall health and longevity.

FIBRE-RICH FOODS

Building your immunity and optimising gut health is achieved by eating fibre and probiotic-rich foods like fruits, vegetables, nuts, seeds, and whole grains. Our gut microbiomes break down the food and extract the nutrients we need. Different foods are broken down by different microbiomes. It's important to fuel your body with many different fibre-rich foods to maintain microbial diversity and overall health. Good gut health also helps signal us to stop eating which naturally helps us to maintain healthy weight without counting calories.

Incorporate fibre-rich foods such as these into your meals and smoothies. Some great options are raspberries, avocadoes, spinach, super greens powder, dates, flaxseed, psyllium husk, oats, and brown rice.

WATER

We are all guilty of overlooking the importance of simply drinking enough water. Your daily water intake goal should be 2.6L for men and 2.1L for women. Water is crucial for healthy digestion, circulation, enhancing nutrient intake, and detoxification. Our skin and organs are made up of cells that contain high amounts of water, and it's important for the hydration of our skin to consume about 2 litres of water every day to make it less prone to dryness and wrinkles.

Sufficient water intake has a direct effect on our energy levels too. By improving the transportation of nutrients to our cells, we feel the benefits of that ongoing source of energy. Try a new morning routine if you're not consuming enough water. The first thing you should do in the morning when you wake up is to drink a half or full bottle of water. After all, you haven't drunk anything for the past eight hours while you were asleep.

TIP: Coconut water or lemon water are natural skin cosmetics. They eliminate toxins and provides vital minerals to hydrate the skin.

DETOXING

The purpose of detoxes is to remove harmful toxins from our blood, organs, muscles, and skin. Purifying our body results in a healthier immune system.

Chia seeds are a powerful detox food that absorb toxins in the digestive system and deposit them in the colon. Chia seeds are virtually tasteless and can easily be added to smoothies and morning oats. Adding lemon juice to your morning glass of water is another fast detox that's easy to do every day. Lemons are a powerful antioxidant that help boost your health and fight disease. However, a lemon drink detox diet alone is not recommended since lemons contain few nutrients and only play a partial role in removing toxins.

Green juices are highly detoxifying and are a good way to consume enough greens (like celery, parsley and leafy greens) for effective results. They provide huge amounts of vitamins, minerals, and antioxidants that flush toxins from your organs, oxygenate the blood, and improve circulation. Ongoing detoxing with loads of greens ultimately means healthy digestion, regular bowel movements, and your best skin complexion.

In summary, the functionality of your digestive system is a major factor that controls the speed of aging and unnecessary inflammation. Foods that include saturated fats and sugar, like fast food, contribute to inflammation and should be avoided. Excess acidity in the body from food like red meat, coffee, and cheese adds to the effects of inflammation. Our cells function better when slightly alkaline and green juices are perfect for achieving this. By subjecting your body to crash diets, your gut becomes sluggish and your body is unable to absorb the nutrients it needs to function. Furthermore, you are undernourishing your skin, hair, muscles, and bones. Once you have the right balance of good gut bacteria, you will benefit from healthy nourishment and energy.

TIPS, TRICKS & SHORTCUTS FOR YOUR LIFESTYLE

Weight management and good health are all about lifestyle. Cooking the right food at home is where you make or break your chances for the fitness and body type that you strive for. Throughout this book you will find that I always encourage you to follow a balanced and calorie-controlled meal plan. The thing that will make cooking and meal preparation successful for you is having the right ingredients and equipment in your kitchen and at your fingertips. The goal here is to take away any anxiety about making decisions about what to eat, how to prepare meals to take to work, and how much food you actually need.

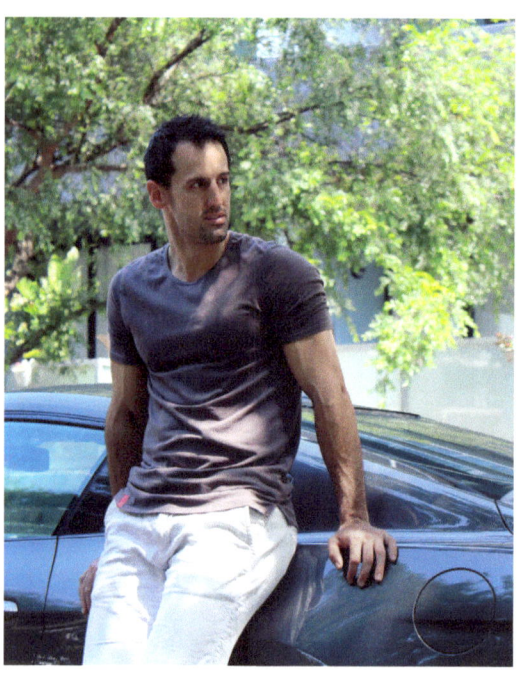

I always aim to cook three to four meals at once. This gives me dinner plus two or three meals for the next day while I'm at work. Remember that you are typically out of the house for about ten hours so be prepared for that. I really hate leaving myself short and not taking food to work because then I'm going to put myself in a position to make a bad decision at lunchtime when I'm hungry. When I prepare my lunch, I graze throughout the day and I don't make bad choices.

A "diet" in many people's understanding of the word is a temporary way to eat. What happens is that people rebound when coming off a diet because they go for the foods that were restricted. Your calorie intake goes up a little and your level of exercise will likely not improve. Diets like this work for a period of time because you cut out the sugar, fat, and calories that you shouldn't have to begin with.

Making an entire lifestyle change to your diet for weight loss is difficult at first. It will be a complete shock to the system. Counting calories won't make sense and your end goal may seem too far away to achieve. Push through this. It is a slow process; be patient. Embrace the journey and keep faith that gradually your results will come. I treat every workout and every meal preparation as a step to next week's workouts and then that week makes me stronger for the week after that. Every week I improve by small percentages, and before I know it, three months have passed and I really see changes in the mirror. This is why setting an endgame is so good. It gives you a deadline and every day is an opportunity to improve. More on this later in chapter 11 - Consistency & Discipline.

The next section describes the tricks I use every single week to help keep me on track with my fitness and physique goals.

- Simple and easy meals can be both delicious and nutritious. I want to cook as quickly as I can at night without missing out on flavour and nutrition. Master just ten recipes and make this easy for yourself.
- Cook in bulk. Preparing several meals at once is obviously time efficient. It's just as simple to make four meals as it is one. Understanding your portion sizes (you'll learn more about this as you read on) will help you in your meal preparations. If you can prepare meals for two days, you'll thank yourself later when you take the following night off from the kitchen.
- Don't retreat. Take a couple of months to double down on learning some cooking basics. This book is your guide to basic meals. Once you know, you know!
- The easiest way to structure your meals is to divide your plate into thirds: ⅓ protein, ⅓ carbs, and ⅓ veggies. This visual guide provides your approximate macronutrient requirements and stops you from overeating.

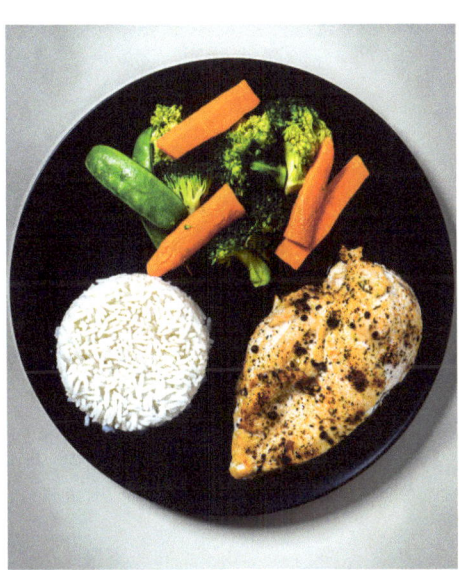

- Read and listen to every source you can to learn about food, diet, and fitness. I've enjoyed hours (make that years) of books and YouTube videos. Then I take what works for me. See references on page 138 for some of my favourite sources.
- Shop one to two times a week. Have food in the house.
- Limit processed food (i.e. anything in packaging or bottles).
- Embrace nutrient-dense food. Seek fresh produce from greengrocers, fresh meat from butchers, and fresh seafood from seafood shops. The quality is far superior to supermarkets.
- Be consistent. Maintain a steady meal plan and eat the same way every day. There is plenty of variety for food, but the structure of meals can remain the same.
- Define your goal. Always have your endgame in mind and chip away at it each day. Improvements will be subtle, so be patient.
- Cheat meals are only okay when you deserve them, not just because it's Sunday. You will naturally cheat when you go out with your friends anyway. Stick to your plan the rest of the week.
- Listen to your body. When your body is tuned in to a good diet with exercise, you instinctively feel what your body needs. Eat when you're hungry and stop when you're full. It's as simple as it sounds.
- Mise en place (me zohn plahs) is French for "putting in place." In professional kitchens, everything you need is set on the bench in front of you before starting to prepare the meal. It makes your time in the kitchen most efficient. For example, the oven is preheated, the ingredients and cooking utensils are set out, and the raw foods are cut and washed as needed.

SEEK VARIETY WITHIN YOUR STRUCTURE

There is no single diet that can be consumed by everyone. Diets vary by country, climate, and culture. Seek variety and experiment with what you like! I refer to "Structure" as making up your meals with the right portion size of protein, carbohydrates, vegetables, and fats. Your body and mind will benefit from a variety of each but you're keeping your meals consistent in size. My shopping list consists primarily of fresh ingredients that are low in sugar and unhealthy fats. I love it because it's easy to shop for each week and I give myself opportunity to stay within my structure.

A way to help hit your macronutrient targets, described in the next chapter, is to make meal preparation a priority rather than always eating for pleasure. We can take some inspiration from studying professional athletes. Athletes need to be on a strict and consistent diet and any deviation from it would have a negative effect on performance. They rely on fixed periods of sleep and frequent intake of food. They are disciplined to stick with their optimal meal plan and their meals are as important as their training. They also need to enjoy what they eat in order to sustain this year after year. If we can adopt a similar mindset to eat the same way consistently, then deciding, *What Should I Eat?* should be a relatively simple choice. We have many food options to rotate through and being consistent is actually manageable and no longer a burden.

Luckily for us, we do not need to be as extreme as professional athletes, so we have opportunity for some indulgence. It just can't be a frequent occurrence in your meal plan.

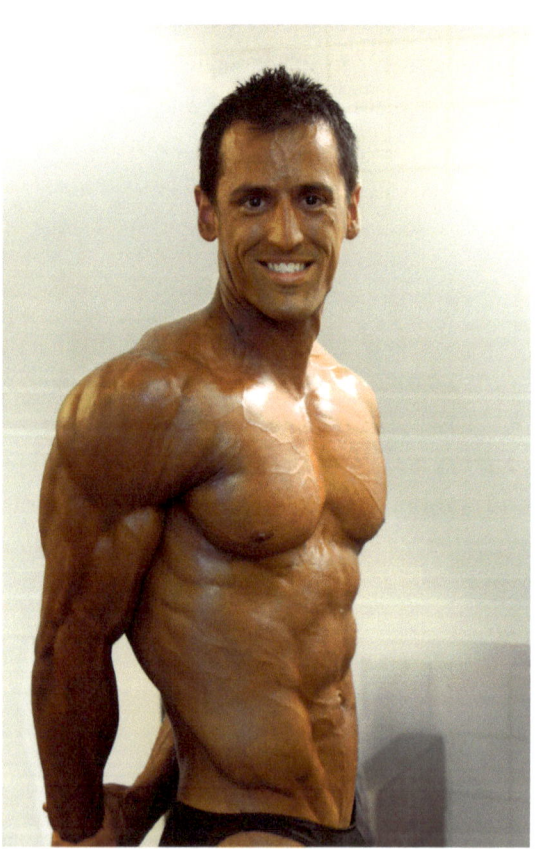

I've experienced firsthand how a strict calorie diet and extreme deprivation can play tricks with your mental state and energy levels. In 2011, I competed in my first body building competition and that strict diet was only manageable for a short time. I really respect anyone who can do this diet to prepare for a body building show. You're at your lowest caloric intake and you're doing the most exercise. Physically you feel terrible, but your body is so beautiful at that point. You look incredible when you're at your worst. Since that experience, I say, a cheat meal like pizza or some chocolate every so often is good for your mind and soul.

MACRONUTRIENTS & CALORIE CALCULATOR TO BUILD YOUR OWN DIET

WEIGHT LOSS VS. WEIGHT GAIN

Everyone has their base metabolic rate (BMR). This is the amount of energy, described in calories, that your body requires simply to function each day. When you add any level of exercise, your daily calorie intake goes up just to maintain your weight.

Weight gain and weight loss is a simple equation. Just remember this golden rule: Calories in (diet) versus calories out (exercise). For weight loss, you need to be in a consistent calorie deficit (below BMR) by a few hundred calories a day. Alternatively, weight gain is a result of excess calories (above BMR) being stored by the body.

Three ways people eat are:

- Low calorie diet with little or no exercise – an unfortunate combination that is not recommended. It's actually unhealthy when you are not consuming your full spectrum of macronutrients and calories. You have little room for error with this approach because your calorie intake has to be extremely precise. The risk to give in to cravings is high because you're low on energy from the restricted calories.
- High calorie diet with extreme exercise – this is the method I subscribe to, but it's certainly not for everyone. It takes a real commitment to hours of exercise each week. For athletes, however, high calorie diets are absolutely crucial to get the necessary fuel for such an active lifestyle.
- A balance of the two – I encourage most people to take this approach. Consume a well-rounded diet that gives your body and mind fuel to be active and fuel for recovery. Do your exercise and participate in activities you enjoy. This is the way to a healthier body. Make it a lifestyle which means you don't even think about it. You just do it.

MY OPINION ON DIETS

In my opinion, losing or maintaining weight is most effectively achieved with a combination of diet and exercise. There are no tricks or special foods for losing weight. Being disciplined and consistent with your meals and exercise is what is actually important, more than the diet you think you need. Being consistent means staying true to your six meals per day, seven days a week, from January through December. If this is new to you then it may not be easy at first and it may take some effort for a few weeks. You need to stick with it to see results and develop your routine until it's not even a thought.

Keep in mind that when you want to align with a particular diet plan, you need to have strict conformity in order for it to work. Diets are normally temporary, so you can go on and off and your weight will yo-yo just the same. I've chosen a lifestyle over the past fifteen years to maintain my weight by balancing good food with daily exercise. The foods that I eat and the foods that you choose to eat in alignment with your macronutrient calorie count become your "diet." The consistency of exercising just thirty minutes a day allows you to eat food without thinking about it too much. I do typically prepare and eat clean food, but when I feel like a cheat meal once in a blue moon, it's not even a thought and it doesn't affect me at all.

It doesn't really matter which diet you want to follow. You shouldn't discriminate against any or strictly favour just one. One isn't superior to the other. Adapt to what works for you and find one that you can stick to. Longevity and understanding the theory should be your goal. The calories you burn through activity will constantly fluctuate each day along with other biological factors going on that we cannot consider. Make minor adjustments accordingly depending on what your body is telling you. Just remember: Calories in (diet) versus calories out (exercise). Be consistent with training and eating.

CALCULATING YOUR BASE METABOLIC RATE

Calculate your BMR using the Harrison Benedict Formula below. Divide your daily BMR, in calories, by the number of meals you eat in the day; this will give you your portion sizes. I follow the traditional method of eating every two to three hours which keeps my metabolism working nicely and I rarely need to deal with cravings. This works out to be about six to seven meals per day. Once you understand portion sizes, overeating shouldn't be a problem. Time to get out your calculator.

The Harrison Benedict Formula

MEN

BMR = 66.5 + (13.75 × weight in kg) + (5.003 × height in cm) - (6.755 × age in years)

WOMEN

BMR = 655.1 + (9.563 × weight in kg) + (1.850 × height in cm) - (4.676 × age in years)

Multiply your BMR by your level of activity:

Little to no exercise, multiply by 1.2
Light exercise a few times a week, multiply by 1.375
Moderate exercise 3–5 times a week, multiply by 1.55
Heavy exercise 6–7 times a week, multiply by 1.725

EXAMPLE

MY STATS

Male / Weight: 90kg / Height: 187cm / Age: 38 / Heavy Exercise
BMR = [66.5 + (13.75 × 90) + (5.003 × 187) − (6.755 × 38)] × 1.725 = 3,420 calories/day
Meal Portion Size = 3,420 calories per day / 7 meals per day = 489 calories per meal

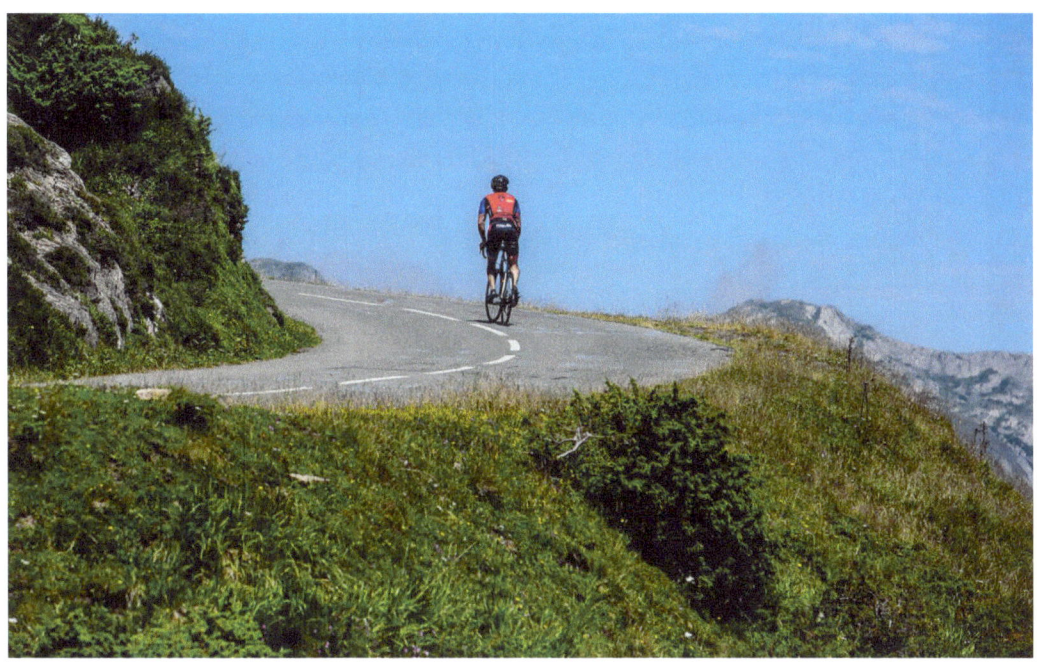

WHAT IS YOUR MACRONUTRIENT BREAKDOWN?

We've worked out how many daily calories you need to maintain weight, taking into account your level of exercise. How do you break that down into protein, carbohydrates, and fats? To quote *The World's Fittest Book* by Ross Edgley, the ratio of protein, carbohydrates, and fats doesn't matter as long as you can stick to it. These are three general ratios to choose from:

High carbohydrate diet:	20% Protein / 70% Carbohydrates / 10% Fats
High fat diet:	20% Protein / 10% Carbohydrates / 70% Fats
Balanced diet:	25% Protein / 50% Carbohydrates / 25% Fats

Let's stick with the balanced diet as the example and breakdown what your daily meal plan needs to look like.

Proteins	4 calories per gram
Carbohydrates	4 calories per gram
Fats	9 calories per gram
Protein:	(3,420 calories × 0.25) / 4 calories per gram / 7 meals per day = 30.5 grams protein per meal
Carbohydrate:	(3,420 calories × 0.5) / 4 calories per gram / 7 meals per day = 61.1 grams carbohydrates per meal
Fats:	(3,420 calories × 0.25) / 9 calories per gram / 7 meals per day = 13.6 grams fat per meal

HOW MUCH OF A CALORIE DEFICIT DO YOU NEED TO LOSE WEIGHT?

I previously mentioned that you need to be in a consistent calorie deficit for weight loss. That's achieved by exercising, restricting what you eat, or ideally a combination of both. In my opinion, losing weight by restricting food alone is the hardest option because you eat little food and there is no room for error. You need to be strict with eating less food than you're used to, and brain fog and lethargy will creep in. It's very hard to maintain this method for too long.

Whichever method you choose, how much of a calorie deficit is enough? It's time to get out your calculator again and count calories. Losing about 0.5kg to 1kg per week has been shown to be safe and sustainable. Let's use an example of 10kg as a weight loss goal over 12 weeks.

Burning 7700 calories = 1kg of weight loss

Burning 7700 calories = 1kg of weight loss (3500 calories = 1 pound of weight loss)
Total calories to burn = 10kg x 7,700 calories per kg = 77,000 calories
Time frame is 12 weeks (84 days) = 77,000 calories / 84 days = 917 calorie deficit per day

There are a few more numbers to consider now. If you're like me and want to eat a little more than your BMR, you need to include more exercise to make up the deficit. If your level of exercise is on the bare minimum side, then you need to make up the deficit with less food.

As an example, my BMR without exercise is approximately 2,380 calories per day and a one-hour gym session burns off around 500 calories. Therefore I need to eat 417 calories less than my BMR and workout in the gym for an hour per day to reach a 917 calorie deficit. Alternatively, I can run 10km over an hour and burn 780 calories. Then I only need to eat 137 calories less than BMR. Another way to manipulate these numbers is to extend your target time frame to 15 weeks which reduces the daily calorie deficit to 733 calories.

Having a heart rate monitor to track your calorie expenditure, a well thought out meal plan, and a daily diary to track results are all equally important. When I dieted for my bodybuilding show in 2011, this is exactly how I monitored my progress and was able to perfectly time my peak physique for the show.

EXAMPLE OF DAILY INTAKE & WEEKLY WORKOUTS

We previously calculated your required calorie intake and the breakdown of proteins, carbohydrates, and fats. We used a general equation, but even this calculation can be fine-tuned to suit your level of activity. Calculating a caloric deficit isn't an exact science and you should monitor your habits in the kitchen and in the gym. You can make adjustments by paying attention to how your body is feeling and checking yourself in the mirror (yes, it is okay to do this). Making small changes could mean reducing portion sizes, increasing your training, or, in my case, I eat re-load meals every few weeks, meaning I have a high calorie meal to restore my energy reserves when I'm in a high-volume training block.

What do all of these macronutrient breakdowns and timing of meals really look like in a meal plan? This is my typical example:

5 am	Breakfast	(~550 calories)
7:30 am	Post-workout protein shake	(~150 calories)
9 am	Post-workout meal	(~650 calories)
12 pm	Lunch	(~650 calories)
3 pm	Snack	(~150 calories)
6 pm	Dinner	(~650 calories)
9 pm	Dessert snack	(~470 calories)
Daily Total:		**~3,270 calories**

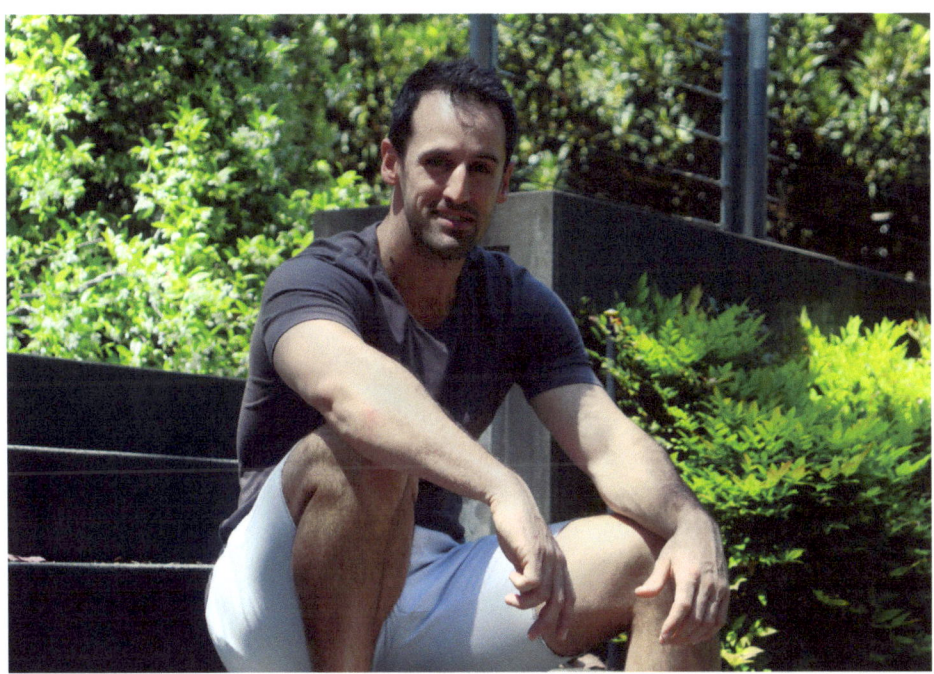

FOOD & WORKOUT DIARY Typical Week - Calories In (FOOD) v Calories Out (EXERCISE)

	SUNDAY	MONDAY	TUESDAY
5AM		Toast x 2 w peanut butter, honey & cinnamon. Greek coffee P 23.6 F 25.5 C 55.3 kcal 545.1	Toast x 2 w peanut butter, honey & cinnamon. Greek coffee P 23.6 F 25.5 C 55.3 kcal 545.1
6AM	1 cup raw oats, mixed berries, protein, honey w water P 43.7 F 12.7 C 102.4 kcal 698.7	WEIGHTS Workout kcal 701.0	WEIGHTS Workout kcal 564.0
7AM			
8AM	10km RUN kcal 783.0	Protein shake P 30 F 2.3 C 3.7 kcal 155.5	Protein shake P 30 F 2.3 C 3.7 kcal 155.5
9AM		250g chicken, 1 cup white rice w brocolli P 60.1 F 4.2 C 57.6 kcal 508.6	200g kangaroo, 1 cup white rice w mixed salad P 43.9 F 4.2 C 62.2 kcal 462.2
10AM	Banana protein pancakes w 5 eggs P 38.5 F 21.9 C 46.5 kcal 537.1	½ celery green juice P 1 F 0.1 C 4.9 kcal 24.5	½ celery green juice P 1 F 0.1 C 4.9 kcal 24.5
11AM			
12PM			
1PM	300g steak w 2 cups potatoes P 71.6 F 47.3 C 63.2 kcal 964.9	250g chicken, 1 cup white rice w brocolli P 60.1 F 4.2 C 57.6 kcal 508.6	200g kangaroo, 1 cup white rice w mixed salad P 43.9 F 4.2 C 62.2 kcal 462.2
2PM		½ celery green juice P 1 F 0.1 C 4.9 kcal 24.5	½ celery green juice P 1 F 0.1 C 4.9 kcal 24.5
3PM			
4PM	200g chicken, 1 cup white rice w veggies P 48.9 F 3.4 C 57.6 kcal 456.6		
5PM		Protein shake P 30 F 2.3 C 3.7 kcal 155.5	Protein shake P 30 F 2.3 C 3.7 kcal 155.5
6PM		1.5km SWIM kcal 390.0	30km BIKE kcal 750.0
7PM	250g chicken, 1 cup white rice w brocolli P 60.1 F 4.2 C 57.6 kcal 508.6	300g salmon, 1 cup white rice, mixed salad P 65.8 F 39.7 C 57.6 kcal 850.9	
8PM			Spagetti bolognase w 200g mince, 1 cup pasta P 50.6 F 13.9 C 88.1 kcal 679.9
9PM	Yogurt w protein powder, berries & musli P 39.5 F 16.1 C 43.9 kcal 478.5	Yogurt w protein powder, berries & musli P 39.5 F 16.1 C 43.9 kcal 478.5	Berry Protein Smoothie P 35.4 F 15.1 C 54 kcal 493.5
10PM			
11PM			
TOTALS	(Drink 3L water) P 302.3 F 105.6 C 371.2 kcal 3644.4	(Drink 2L water) P 311.1 F 94.5 C 289.2 kcal 3251.7	(Drink 2L water) P 259.4 F 67.7 C 339 kcal 3002.9
	Required Daily Calorie Intake kcal 3420.0 Consumed Calories (3644.4) - Required Calories (3420) Surplus/Deficit kcal 224.4	Required Daily Calorie Intake kcal 3420.0 Consumed Calories (3251.7) - Required Calories (3420) Surplus/Deficit kcal -168.3	Required Daily Calorie Intake kcal 3420.0 Consumed Calories (3002.9) - Required Calories (3420) Surplus/Deficit kcal -417.1

WEDNESDAY	THURSDAY	FRIDAY	SATURDAY
Toast x 2 w peanut butter, honey & cinnamon. Greek coffee P 23.6 F 25.5 C 55.3 kcal 545.1		Toast x 2 w peanut butter, honey & cinnamon. Greek coffee P 23.6 F 25.5 C 55.3 kcal 545.1	Toast x 2 w peanut butter, honey & cinnamon. Greek coffee P 23.6 F 25.5 C 55.3 kcal 545.1
1.6km SWIM kcal 416.0	1 cup raw oats, mixed protein, berries, honey w water P 43.7 F 12.7 C 102.4 kcal 698.7	WEIGHTS Workout kcal 449.0	50-90km BIKE kcal 1987.0
Banana Protein Smoothie P 49.4 F 21.3 C 80.4 kcal 710.9		Protein shake P 30 F 2.3 C 3.7 kcal 155.5	
	200g tuna, 1 cup brown rice w ½ avocado P 50.3 F 45.8 C 61.1 kcal 857.8	250g pork, 1 cup white rice w chimmijurri P 64.8 F 11.1 C 69.2 kcal 635.9	
Spagetti bolagnase w 200g mince, 1 cup pasta P 50.6 F 13.9 C 88.1 kcal 679.9	½ celery green juice P 1 F 0.1 C 4.9 kcal 24.5		Banana Protein Smoothie P 49.4 F 21.3 C 80.4 kcal 710.9
			Scrambled eggs x 6 w mushrooms, chilli, avocado on toast P 49.4 F 49.4 C 28.4 kcal 755.8
Spagetti bolagnase w 200g mince, 1 cup pasta P 50.6 F 13.9 C 88.1 kcal 679.9		250g pork, 1 cup white rice w chimmijurri P 64.8 F 11.1 C 69.2 kcal 635.9	
	200g tuna, 1 cup white rice w ½ avocado P 50.3 F 45.8 C 61.1 kcal 857.8		
	½ celery green juice P 1 F 0.1 C 4.9 kcal 24.5		BBQ chicken 200g sandwiches x 2 w salad. Orange & apple juice P 69.4 F 15 C 47 kcal 600.6
		Protein shake P 30 F 2.3 C 3.7 kcal 155.5	
½ cup raw oats, mixed berries, protein, honey w water P 21.9 F 6.7 C 51.7 kcal 354.7	Protein shake P 30 F 2.3 C 3.7 kcal 155.5		
		DINNER OUT P 40 F 30 C 100 kcal 830.0	Ocean trout 200g w prawns 100g & chimmijurri, 1 cup white rice P 66.9 F 21.5 C 69.2 kcal 737.9
	250g pork, 1 cup white rice w chimmijurri P 64.8 F 11.1 C 69.2 kcal 635.9		
Fried rice 1 cup with prawns 100g P 34.6 F 16.7 C 59.9 kcal 528.3			
			Chocolate/Peanut Butter Cups P 2.7 F 10 C 5 kcal 120.8
Yogurt w protein powder, berries & musli P 39.5 F 16.1 C 43.9 kcal 478.5	Yogurt w protein powder, berries & musli P 39.5 F 16.1 C 43.9 kcal 478.5	Berries Protein Smoothie P 35.4 F 15.1 C 54 kcal 493.5	
(Drink 2L water) P 270.2 F 114.1 C 467.4 kcal 3977.3	(Drink 2L water) P 280.6 F 134 C 351.2 kcal 3733.2	(Drink 2L water) P 288.6 F 97.4 C 355.1 kcal 3451.4	(Drink 3L water) P 261.4 F 142.7 C 285.3 kcal 3471.1
Required Daily Calorie Intake kcal 3420.0 Consumed Calories (3977.3) - Required Calories (3420) Surplus/Deficit kcal 557.3	Required Daily Calorie Intake kcal 3420.0 Consumed Calories (3733.2) - Required Calories (3420) Surplus/Deficit kcal 313.2	Required Daily Calorie Intake kcal 3420.0 Consumed Calories (3451.4) - Required Calories (3420) Surplus/Deficit kcal 31.4	Required Daily Calorie Intake kcal 3420.0 Consumed Calories (3471.1) - Required Calories (3420) Surplus/Deficit kcal 51.1

BUILD YOUR OWN MEAL PLAN Typical Week - Calories In v Calories Out

	SUNDAY	MONDAY	TUESDAY
5AM	P F C kcal	P F C kcal	P F C kcal
6AM	P F C kcal	P F C kcal	P F C kcal
7AM	P F C kcal	P F C kcal	P F C kcal
8AM	P F C kcal	P F C kcal	P F C kcal
9AM	P F C kcal	P F C kcal	P F C kcal
10AM	P F C kcal	P F C kcal	P F C kcal
11AM	P F C kcal	P F C kcal	P F C kcal
12PM	P F C kcal	P F C kcal	P F C kcal
1PM	P F C kcal	P F C kcal	P F C kcal
2PM	P F C kcal	P F C kcal	P F C kcal
3PM	P F C kcal	P F C kcal	P F C kcal
4PM	P F C kcal	P F C kcal	P F C kcal
5PM	P F C kcal	P F C kcal	P F C kcal
6PM	P F C kcal	P F C kcal	P F C kcal
7PM	P F C kcal	P F C kcal	P F C kcal
8PM	P F C kcal	P F C kcal	P F C kcal
9PM	P F C kcal	P F C kcal	P F C kcal
10PM	P F C kcal	P F C kcal	P F C kcal
11PM	P F C kcal	P F C kcal	P F C kcal
TOTALS	(Drink 2L water) P F C kcal Required Daily Calorie Intake kcal Consumed Calories - Required Calories Surplus/Deficit kcal	(Drink 2L water) P F C kcal Required Daily Calorie Intake kcal Consumed Calories - Required Calories Surplus/Deficit kcal	(Drink 2L water) P F C kcal Required Daily Calorie Intake kcal Consumed Calories - Required Calories Surplus/Deficit kcal

What Should I Eat?

WEDNESDAY	THURSDAY	FRIDAY	SATURDAY
P .... F .... C .... kcal	P .... F .... C .... kcal	P .... F .... C .... kcal	P .... F .... C .... kcal ....
P .... F .... C .... kcal	P .... F .... C .... kcal	P .... F .... C .... kcal	P .... F .... C .... kcal ....
P .... F .... C .... kcal	P .... F .... C .... kcal	P .... F .... C .... kcal	P .... F .... C .... kcal ....
P .... F .... C .... kcal	P .... F .... C .... kcal	P .... F .... C .... kcal	P .... F .... C .... kcal ....
P .... F .... C .... kcal	P .... F .... C .... kcal	P .... F .... C .... kcal	P .... F .... C .... kcal ....
P .... F .... C .... kcal	P .... F .... C .... kcal	P .... F .... C .... kcal	P .... F .... C .... kcal ....
P .... F .... C .... kcal	P .... F .... C .... kcal	P .... F .... C .... kcal	P .... F .... C .... kcal ....
P .... F .... C .... kcal	P .... F .... C .... kcal	P .... F .... C .... kcal	P .... F .... C .... kcal ....
P .... F .... C .... kcal	P .... F .... C .... kcal	P .... F .... C .... kcal	P .... F .... C .... kcal ....
P .... F .... C .... kcal	P .... F .... C .... kcal	P .... F .... C .... kcal	P .... F .... C .... kcal ....
P .... F .... C .... kcal	P .... F .... C .... kcal	P .... F .... C .... kcal	P .... F .... C .... kcal ....
P .... F .... C .... kcal	P .... F .... C .... kcal	P .... F .... C .... kcal	P .... F .... C .... kcal ....
P .... F .... C .... kcal	P .... F .... C .... kcal	P .... F .... C .... kcal	P .... F .... C .... kcal ....
P .... F .... C .... kcal	P .... F .... C .... kcal	P .... F .... C .... kcal	P .... F .... C .... kcal ....
P .... F .... C .... kcal	P .... F .... C .... kcal	P .... F .... C .... kcal	P .... F .... C .... kcal ....
P .... F .... C .... kcal	P .... F .... C .... kcal	P .... F .... C .... kcal	P .... F .... C .... kcal ....
P .... F .... C .... kcal	P .... F .... C .... kcal	P .... F .... C .... kcal	P .... F .... C .... kcal ....
P .... F .... C .... kcal	P .... F .... C .... kcal	P .... F .... C .... kcal	P .... F .... C .... kcal ....
(Drink 2L water) P .... F .... C .... kcal	(Drink 2L water) P .... F .... C .... kcal	(Drink 2L water) P .... F .... C .... kcal	(Drink 2L water) P .... F .... C .... kcal ....
Required Daily Calorie Intake .... kcal Consumed Calories .... - Required Calories .... Surplus/Deficit .... kcal	Required Daily Calorie Intake .... kcal Consumed Calories .... - Required Calories .... Surplus/Deficit .... kcal	Required Daily Calorie Intake .... kcal Consumed Calories .... - Required Calories .... Surplus/Deficit .... kcal	Required Daily Calorie Intake .... kcal Consumed Calories .... - Required Calories .... Surplus/Deficit .... kcal

WORKOUT DIARY & BMR CALORIE COUNT Typical Week

	SUNDAY		MONDAY		TUESDAY	
WEIGHTS			WEIGHTS	701	WEIGHTS	564
AEROBIC	10km RUN	783	1.5km SWIM	390	30km BIKE	750
TOTAL		783		1,091		1,314
ACTUAL BMR (DAILY)	2379 + 783 = 3162 calories		2379 + 1091 = 3470 calories		2379 + 1314 = 3693 calories	

We previously calculated our Base Metabolic Rate using the Harrison Benedict formula which is the minimum number of calories that our body requires daily to function and maintain weight.

The above table is a record of my typical training week and my calorie expenditure. As you can see, my actual daily BMR fluctuates quite considerably. Over the course of the week, it averages out almost exactly as calculated by the formula. See across on page 35.

As an exercise, it's interesting for me to keep track of myself from time to time and compare what I'm actually doing versus what I set out in a meal plan on paper. To re-iterate the message on page 29, while counting calories is important starting out, you should monitor your habits in the kitchen and in the gym with diaries like this.

Don't stress if one day you're in a calorie surplus, you just need to get on track the follow day. Over time, calorie counting becomes intuitive but I do recommend recording your food intake and exercise like this if weight management is important to you to learn. The goal here is to keep ourselves accountable and consistent over the long term.

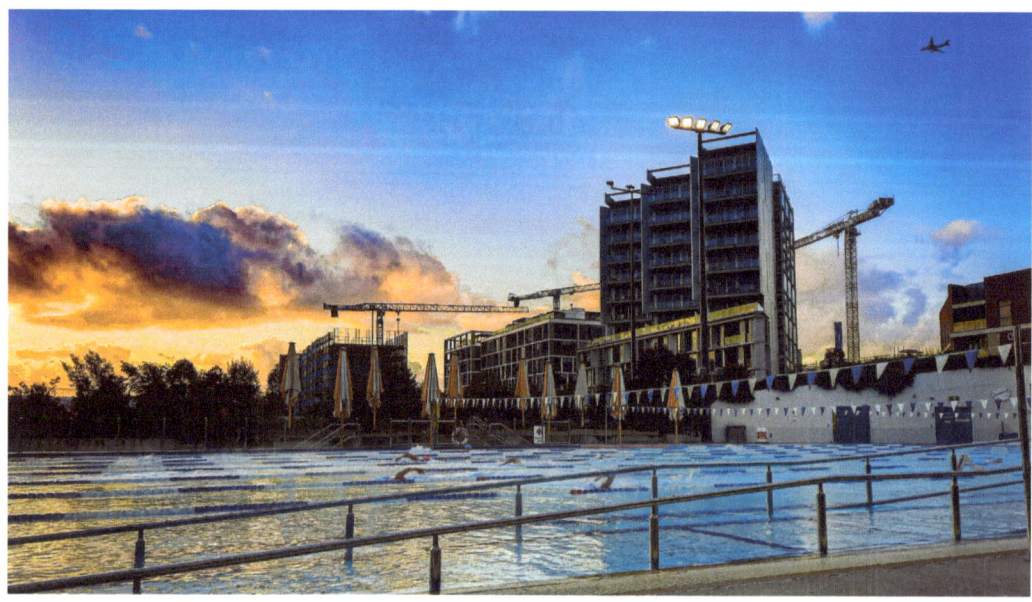

WEDNESDAY		THURSDAY		FRIDAY		SATURDAY	
1.6km SWIM	416	REST DAY		WEIGHTS	449	90km BIKE	1,987
	416		0		449		1,987
2379 + 416 = 2795 calories		2379 calories		2379 + 449 = 2828 calories		2379 + 1987 = 4366 calories	

ACTUAL BMR

AVERAGE REQUIRED DAILY CALORIE INTAKE

(Base Calories (2379kcal) + Exercise Calories)/7 days   3242

CALCULATED BMR

REQUIRED DAILY CALORIE INTAKE   3420

Calculating calories is not an exact science but still, it's a close estimate.
Adjust as necessary to suit your activity level.

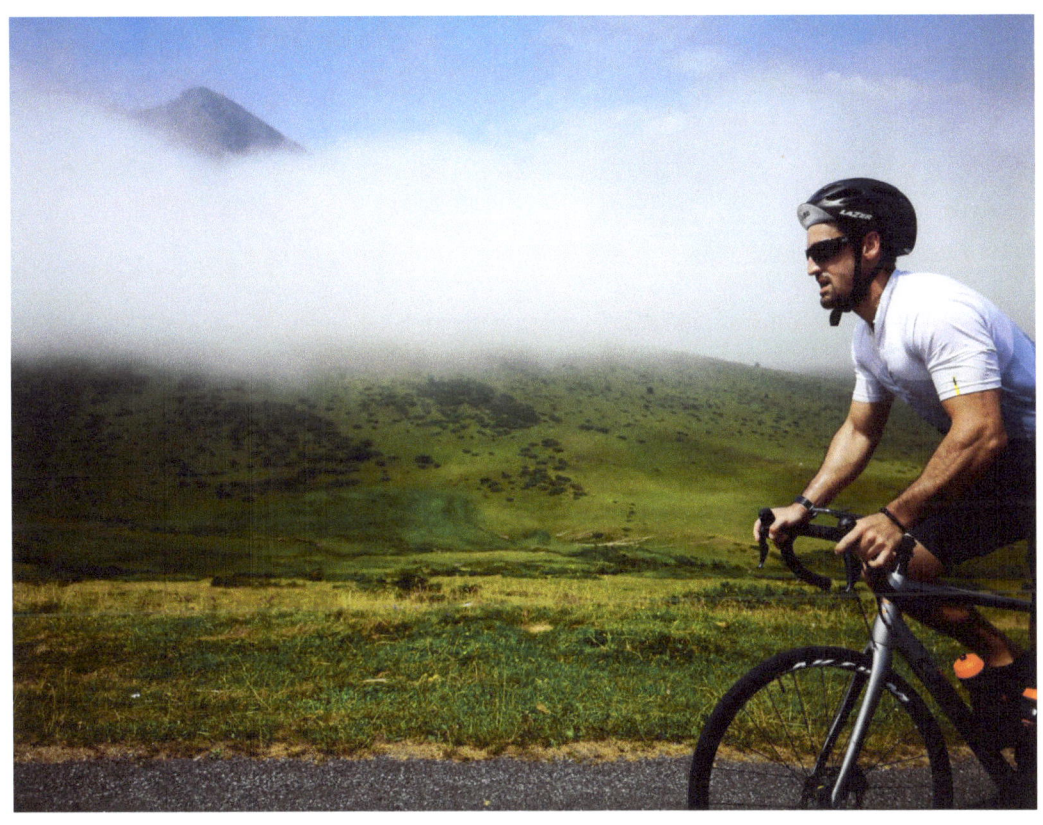

What Should I Eat? 35

CONSISTENCY & DISCIPLINE

Consistency and discipline go hand in hand. Your motivation to stay consistent with cooking your meals is your decision alone. We all have different reasons for succeeding in the gym and the kitchen. For me, my motivation is that I like being able to compete in high-performance events which depend on good nutrition. Competing gives me a sense of identity, and I like the journey to prepare for competition day. There are months of learning, training, and sacrifice to get into my best shape. I get an amazing feeling of achievement when I've finished an event and it's a high that I continue to chase. I've committed to my health and fitness for nearly 20 years and I don't want to see it slip away by becoming complacent.

Being consistent with your nutrition is the key to longevity and truly seeing (and maintaining) results in your health and physique. It's important to experiment in the kitchen and find creative ways to nourish yourself and your family so you don't get bored and resort to eating foods that aren't good for you. There's no point in looking good if you are actually unhealthy. Fad diets can do more harm than good and will catch up with you eventually. They're just a temporary fix until you lose weight or feel fit again, and they aren't sustainable. I don't see the logic in denying yourself certain foods because it's only going to lead to cravings, bad choices, and rebounding back to where you started.

I've found that a balanced approach works for me over the long term, whereby I take in a significant variety of fresh produce and proteins, maintain carbohydrates and fats, and graze throughout the day. Over time and with a lot of trial and error, I have my diet dialled in. My energy levels stay high and I know exactly when and how much I should eat before and after workouts and while I'm at work. I believe I have been successful in keeping my health and immunity relatively high and I don't often get sick. This allows me to keep training, working, and competing. I've tried different diets such as intermittent fasting where you only eat during a certain time of day, low sugar diets, and restricting carbohydrates at night, thinking this would keep me lean. I didn't feel good following these methods and found the approach that works for me. I encourage you to try all of these diets and if one of them suits you then stick with it. The same goes for the meals you eat.

"You are far more powerful than your own mind allows you to believe. That's not just a throwaway comment, it's legit."
– Adventurer Ross Edgley

To create a meal plan, you really only need to be able to make ten meals, a few smoothies, and a couple of snacks. Since I've been cooking with a larger repertoire of meals, I enjoy rotating meals in and out of my nutrition plan while still achieving my macronutrient targets. This has played a huge part of my performance and physique success. Being patient is key as well; I think three months is a good time frame to make any sort of transformation. It's gradual and you should manage your expectation that you might be in it for the long haul. Time is going to pass anyway, so try and chip away at learning a little about food as you go.

Learning to cook and adopt a certain way of eating isn't going to be an overnight success. Set your goal, whether it's to learn new recipes or start paying attention to portion sizes. Trying to diet and get on a 12-week fitness plan may see you slide backwards at some point. If that happens, it's okay; just get right back to your plan. Hopefully after a few months you've developed the right habits to continue year after year. Your goal should be to understand sufficiently how the food you eat affects your health and weight. The habits you develop will become automatic and counting calories won't be something you need to worry about anymore.

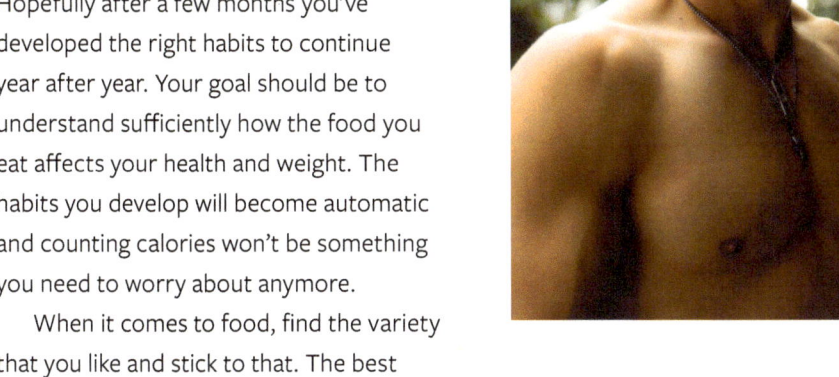

When it comes to food, find the variety that you like and stick to that. The best diet plan, with the nutritionals and macros all worked out on paper, will be useless if you can't maintain it in real life. Lifestyle and meal plans have to be a balance between optimal nutrition and what's enjoyable as a human. Stick within the calorie structure outlined in this book and there's your meal plan.

Discipline is what keeps you on track on those days when you really don't want to exercise or stick to your meal plan. Choosing a lifestyle that suits you is probably the best thing you can do. Decide how much exercise you can do and then figure out your meal sizes as outlined in chapter 9 - Macronutrients & Calorie Calculator. There isn't really an off season. Ever. It has to be that way. The days when you really don't want to cook or train are the days you absolutely have to. Ironically, these training sessions are usually the best ones. When you see some success it will give you to confidence to keep going. Give yourself time to get there; there's no need to judge yourself against other people. My level of health, fitness, and cooking ability may be above some people, but I'm a long way behind a lot of other people and they're a long way behind someone else too. The important thing is that you're happy with what you can manage for your lifestyle.

"Doing what you hate to do but doing it like you love it. You give up on the slightest struggle without discipline." – Mike Tyson

SUMMARY

MAKE WAY FOR NEW THINKING

We covered quite a few topics in preparing you to become capable in the kitchen and get you thinking about how best to nourish yourself and family. I've come to realise that my lifestyle and nutrition is as much to do with how I think and approach my diet as it is to do with cooking my meals.

In summary:

- Embrace the journey of learning new cooking skills rather than thinking about it as a chore.
- Making the mental shift for taking control of your nutrition is challenging at first. Your true motivation and purpose for eating right over the long term is your decision alone.
- There isn't one single diet that best suits everyone. Experiment with an approach and macronutrient percentages that leave you full and satisfied without risking your weight.
- Your meal plan doesn't need to be complicated so try to not get overwhelmed with it all. Learn to make a few meals, smoothies and snacks well and you're covered.
- Patience is key. Any sort of transformation is gradual so chip away at it day by day. Three months is a reasonable time frame to see new habits develop.
- Lifestyle and meal plans have to be a balance between optimal nutrition and what's enjoyable as a human.
- Discipline is what keeps you on track. The days when you really don't want to cook or train are the days you absolutely have to.

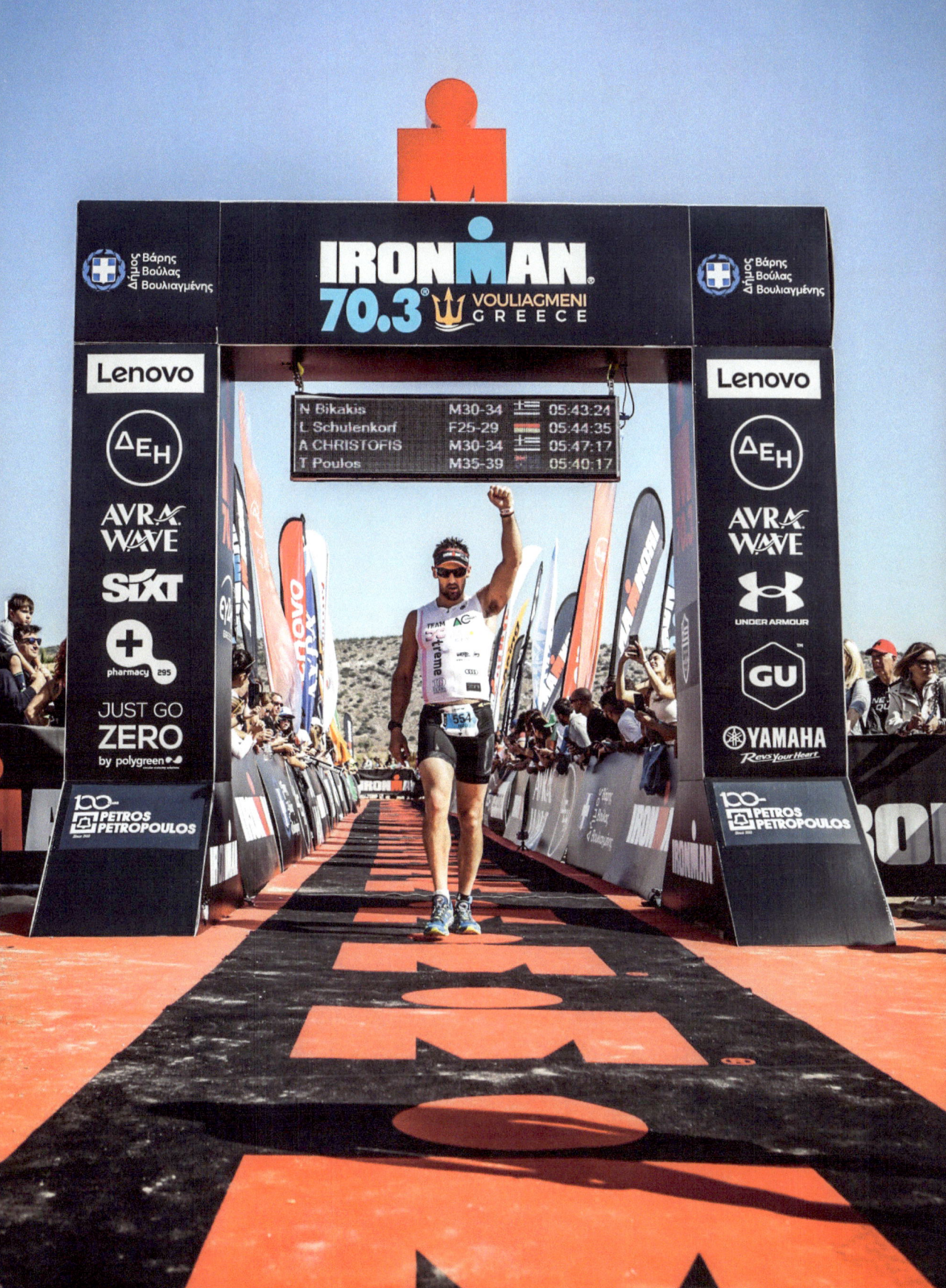

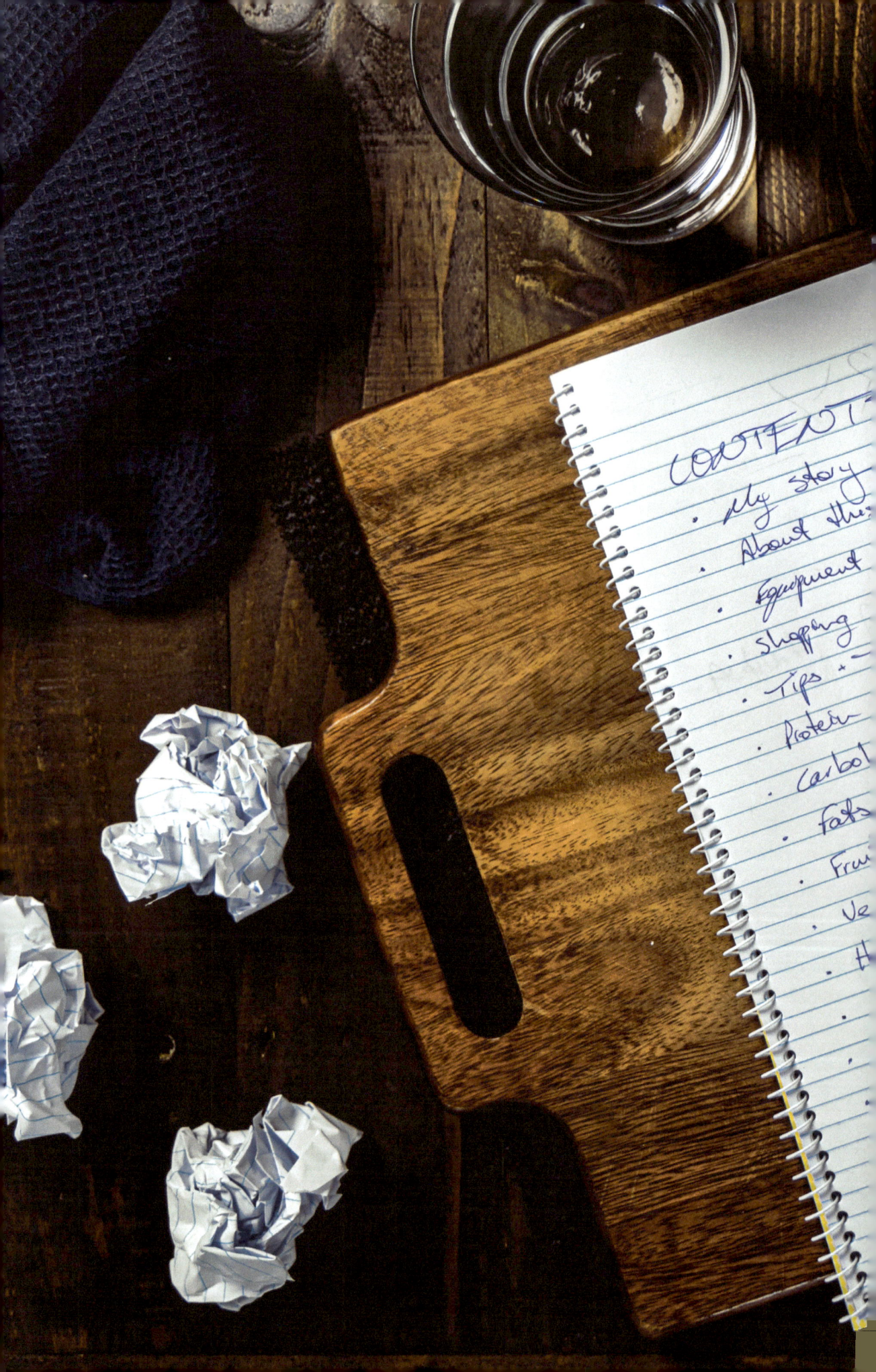

SCRAMBLED EGGS with herbs

	P	C	F	kcal
5 eggs	33	0	25.8	363.8
1 tbs milk	0.7	1.3	0.7	14.3
1 tbs olive oil	0	0	13.7	123.3
4 mushrooms	1.1	1.2	0	9.2
1 small chilli	0.6	1.9	0	10
1 tsp basil + parsley	0	0	0	0
2 slices sourdough	12.4	23.5	5.9	196.7
½ avocado	1.6	0.5	17.0	161.4
1 serving	49.4g	28.4g	63.1g	879.1 kcal

BREAKFAST

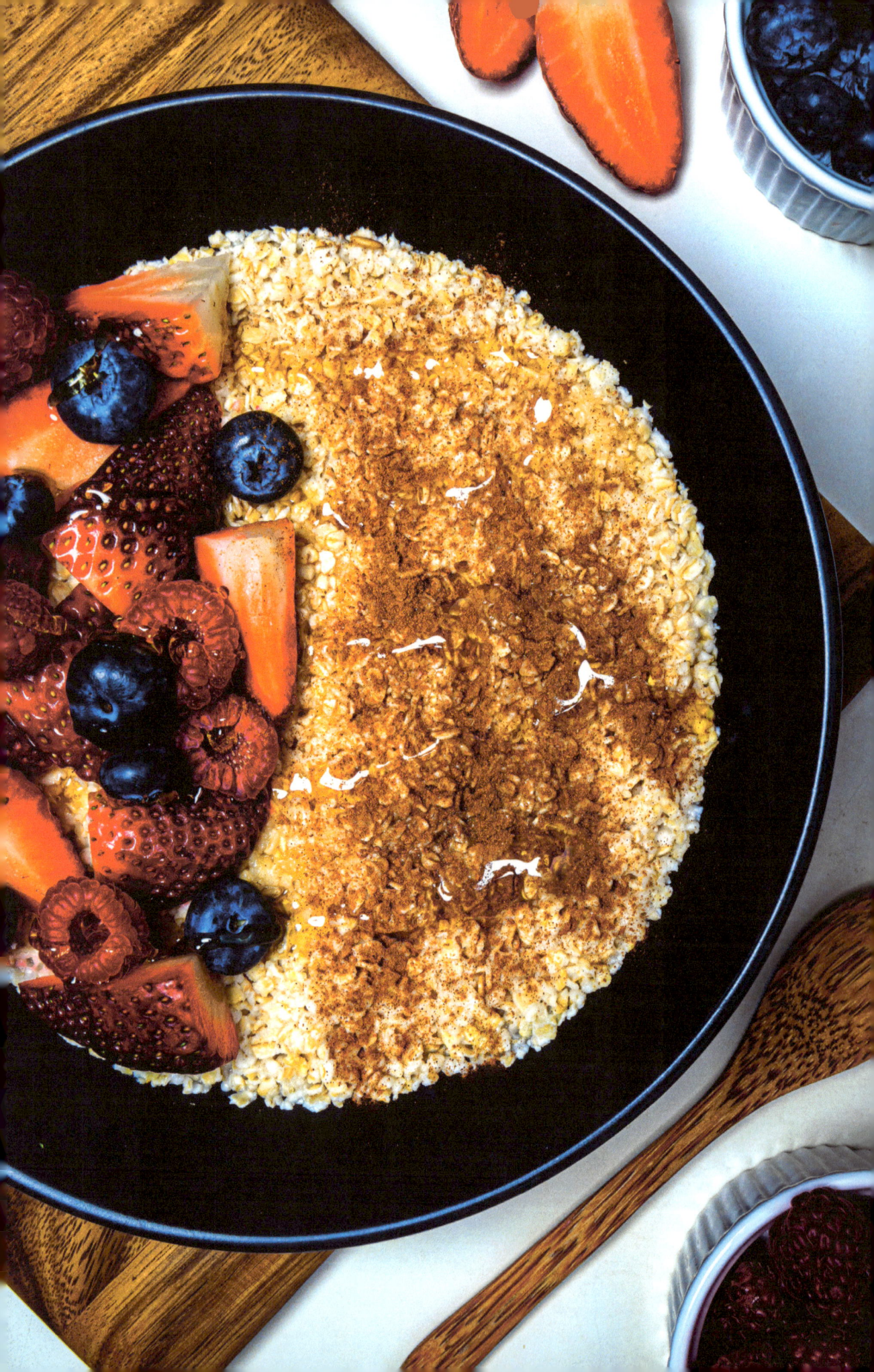

OATS & BERRIES WITH PROTEIN POWDER

This has to be the fastest, cheapest, and easiest snack that covers your nutritional bases. When I have 2 minutes to pack a meal, I turn to oats & protein powder. Remember that our meals are not always going to be glamorous but this is something tasty and your carbs, protein, and antioxidants are all covered!

PREP : 3 MINUTES | COOK : 1 MINUTE | SERVES : 1

1 cup quick oats

1 scoop whey protein

½ cup mixed berries

1 tbs honey

Cinnamon (optional)

Mix the oats, whey protein, and berries in your bowl.

Add boiling water just to cover the oats.

Microwave for 30 seconds and repeat once more. Microwaving for longer than 30 seconds at a time can cause the oats to bubble over (I learnt that the hard way).

Serve with a drizzle of honey and a sprinkle of cinnamon, if desired.

CALORIES 689.7KCAL | PROTEIN 43.7G | CARBS 101.5G | FATS 12.1G

Peanut Butter & Honey Toast with Banana & Cinnamon

A great kick-start to your day. This is full of energy and ideal for breakfast or as a pre-workout snack. Opt for natural peanut butter with no added sugar or additives, only the nutrients from peanuts.

PREP : 10 MINUTES | COOK : 0 MINUTES | SERVES : 1

2 slices sourdough or multigrain bread

2 tbs peanut butter

1 banana

1 tbs honey

½ tsp cinnamon

Toast your favourite sourdough or multigrain bread.

Spread on a generous amount of peanut butter.

Slice your banana and place on top of the peanut butter.

Drizzle honey over the top.

Finally, sprinkle a small amount of cinnamon over the toast. Too much can be overpowering.

> The benefit of peanut butter for breakfast, or snacks at any time, is that it stabilizes blood sugar levels which means you have sustained energy and you won't feel starved and give in to food cravings.

CALORIES 612.4KCAL | PROTEIN 24.3G | CARBS 71.2G | FATS 25.6G

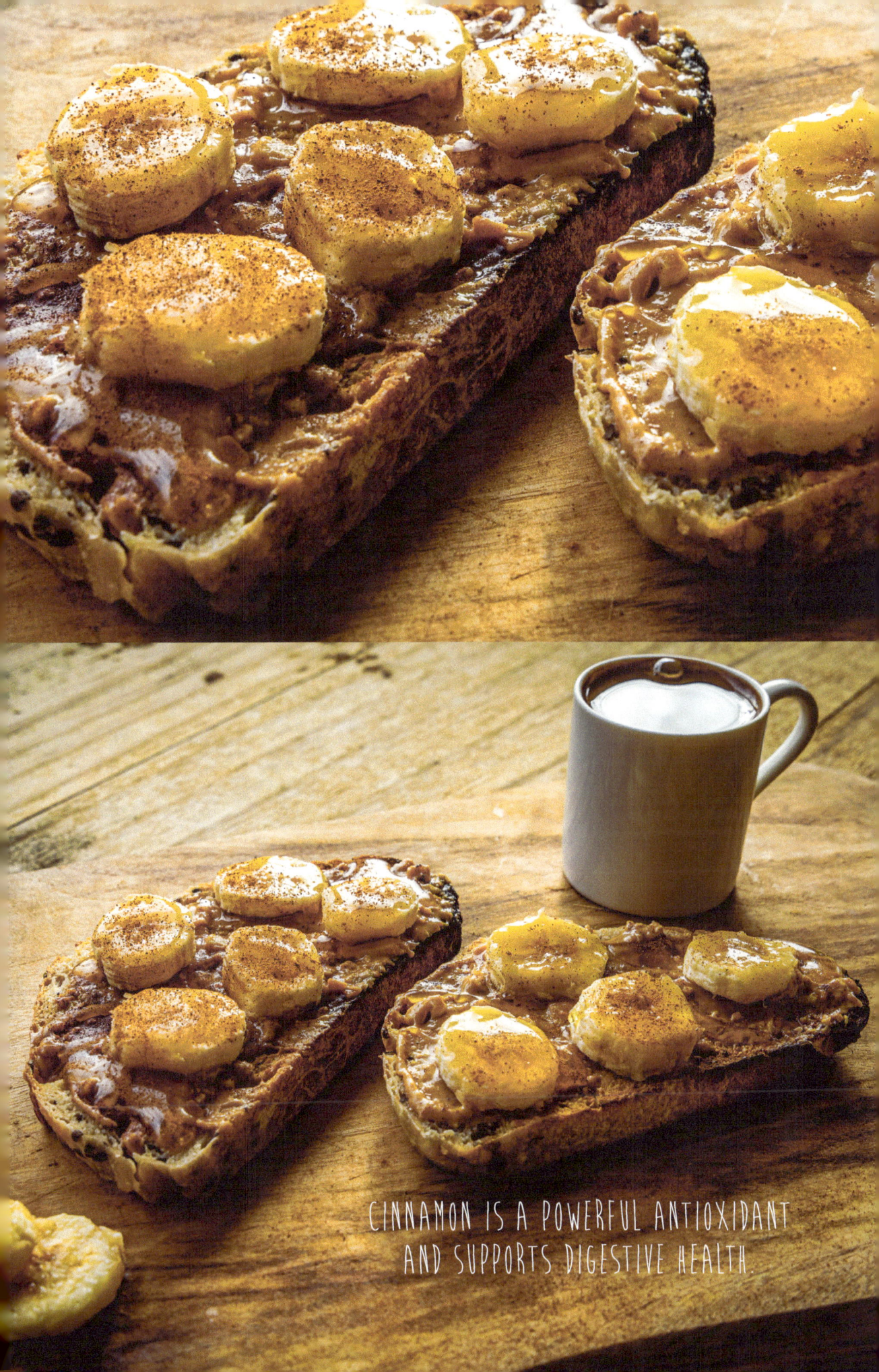

Cinnamon is a powerful antioxidant and supports digestive health.

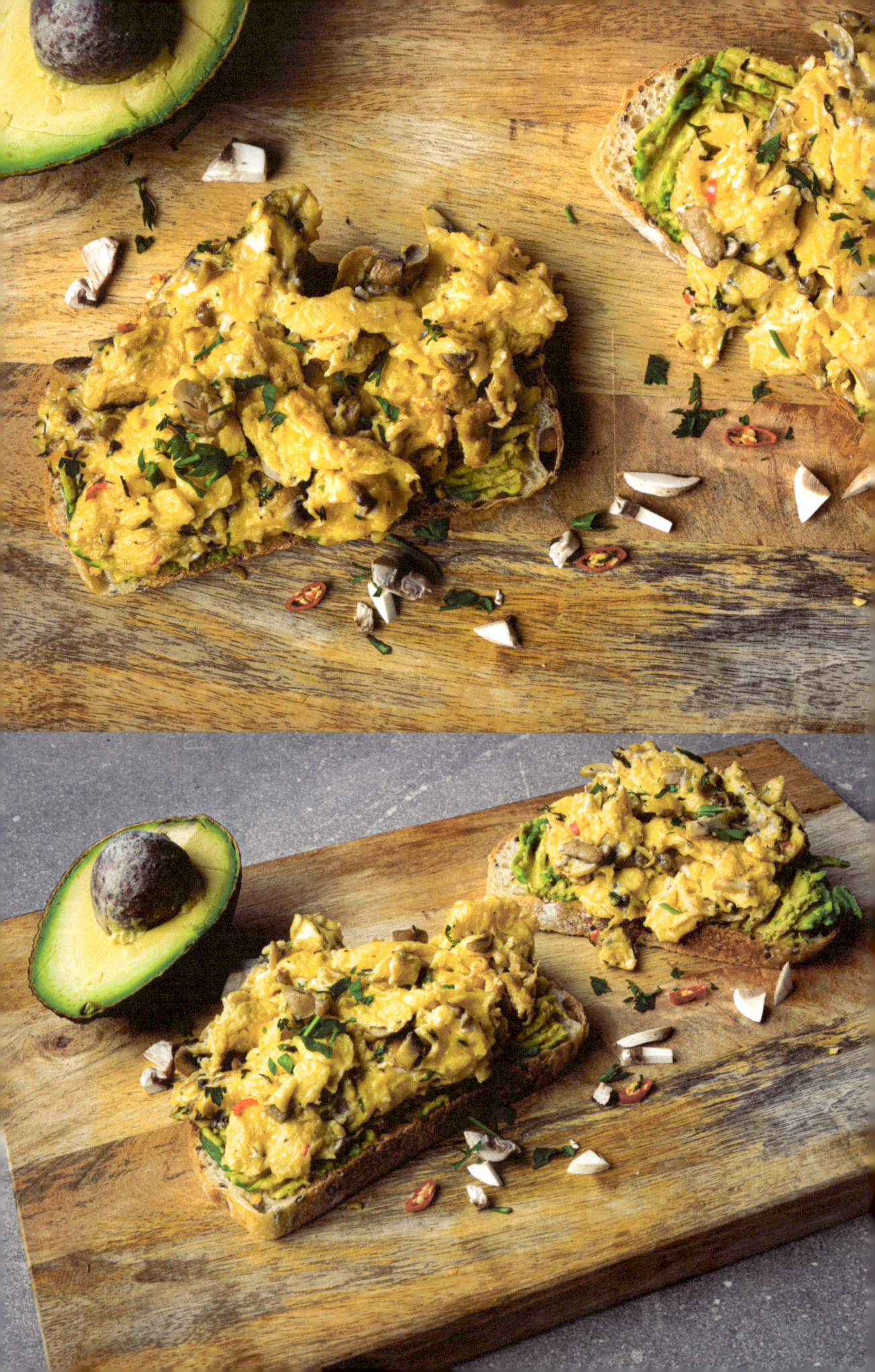

SCRAMBLED EGGS WITH CHILLI, MUSHROOMS & HERBS

Scrambled eggs can be just scrambled eggs, or you can make them into a complete meal. Serve with toast, avocado, and herbs to get your carbs, fats, and antioxidants into your meal. The trick with scrambled eggs is to cook them over low heat and keep moving them around the pan. Fold the eggs as you cook to give it some shape.

PREP : 10 MINUTES | COOK : 10 MINUTES | SERVES : 1

5 eggs

1–2 tbs milk

1 tbs olive oil for cooking

4 mushrooms, finely chopped

1 small chilli, finely chopped

1 tsp freshly chopped basil and/or parsley

2 slices sourdough bread, toasted

½ avocado

Pinch of salt & pepper (optional)

Crack the eggs in a bowl and add a splash of milk. (A small amount of milk will give the eggs more volume.) Whisk with a fork.

Heat the olive oil in the pan on low to medium heat. Add the mushrooms and chilli and cook for a minute.

Pour the egg mixture into the pan with the mushrooms and chilli. After 30 seconds, start moving the eggs around with a flat spatula or wooden spoon.

Sprinkle the herbs into the eggs and keep stirring them until the eggs reach your desired consistency.

Serve on sourdough toast with a spread of avocado. Add salt & pepper if desired.

Eggs are high in healthy fats and have several health benefits, including supporting brain function. The fat content and vitamins are in the yolks; egg whites have no fat at all. If you're looking to lower the calorie count regardless, limit your egg yolks.

CALORIES 879.1KCAL | PROTEIN 49.4G | CARBS 28.4G | FATS 63.1G

Banana & Protein Pancakes with Berries

These pancakes are packed with protein and healthy calories. The mixture is similar to a banana smoothie (see page 124), and the pancakes are naturally sweetened with the addition of mixed berries and some honey. It's a perfect meal any time of the day when you want that sweet hit.

PREP : 5 MINUTES | COOK : 10–15 MINUTES | SERVES : 2

5 eggs

1 banana

1 scoop whey protein

½ cup rolled oats

1 tsp greens superfood powder

1–2 tbs peanut butter

1 tsp cocoa powder

1 tsp psyllium husk

1 tbs olive oil for cooking

½ cup mixed berries

1 tbs honey

1 tsp cinnamon

Add the eggs, banana, protein, oats, peanut butter, cocoa, and psyllium husk to your bullet blender and blend thoroughly. It will be a thick mixture.

Heat the olive oil in the pan on medium heat.

Pour the pancake mixture into your pan. For the best presentation, make 4 to 6 smaller pancakes. If you're low on time or are serving just yourself, one large, badly flipped pancake that fills the pan will do.

Cook until the mixture becomes firm. Flip once.

Plate up with your choice of berries, such as raspberries, blueberries, and/or strawberries.

Drizzle honey over your pancake and sprinkle a small amount of cinnamon over it for extra sweetener.

The thick consistency of the mixture comes from the eggs. This isn't a traditional pancake batter with flour, so don't be shy to add extras to the mix, like dates and superfood powders.

FOR PICTURE PERFECT PANCAKES, ADD ½ TSP BAKING SODA TO THE MIXTURE.

CALORIES 660.4KCAL | PROTEIN 38.5G | CARBS 45.6G | FATS 35.6G

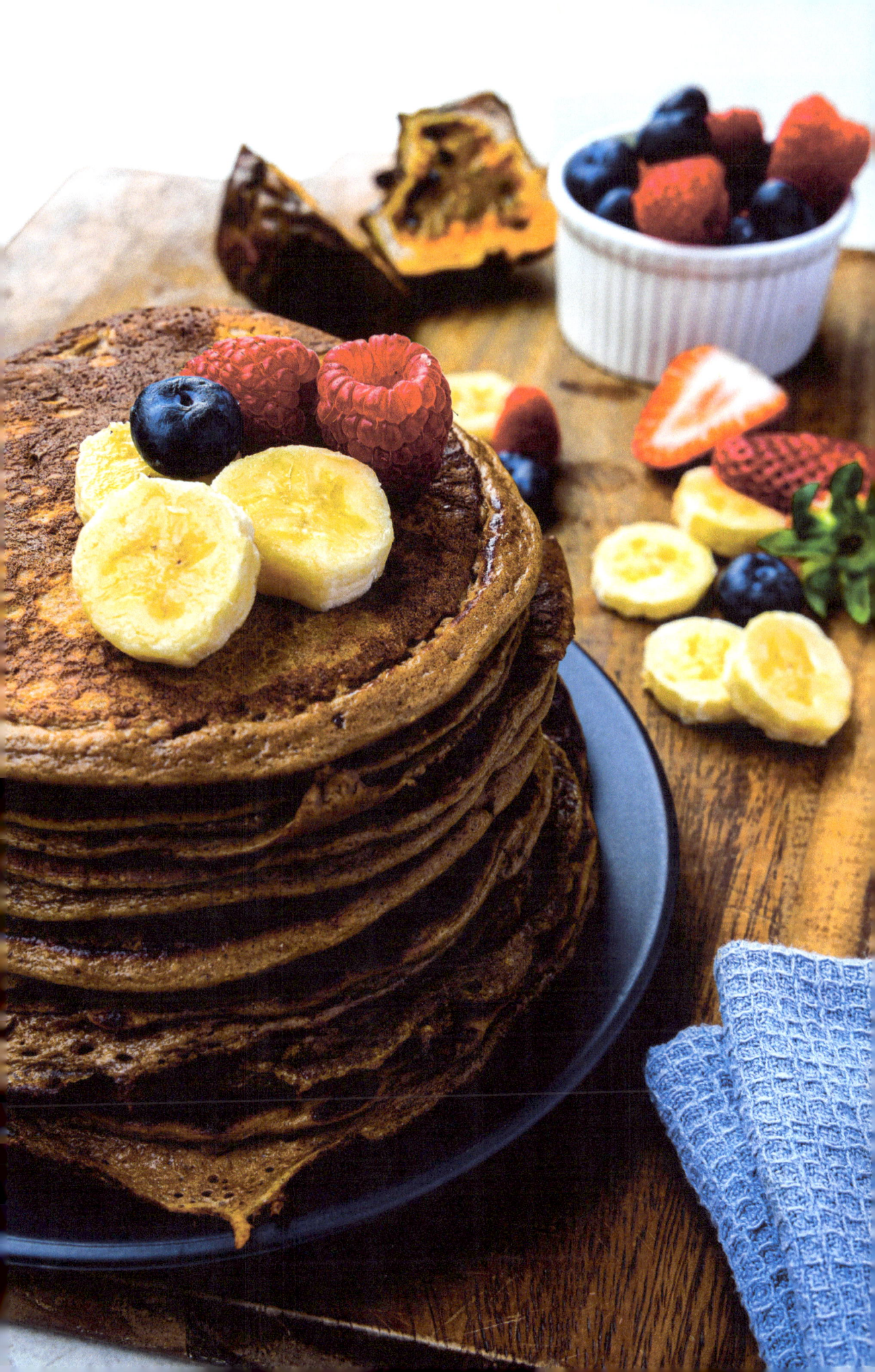

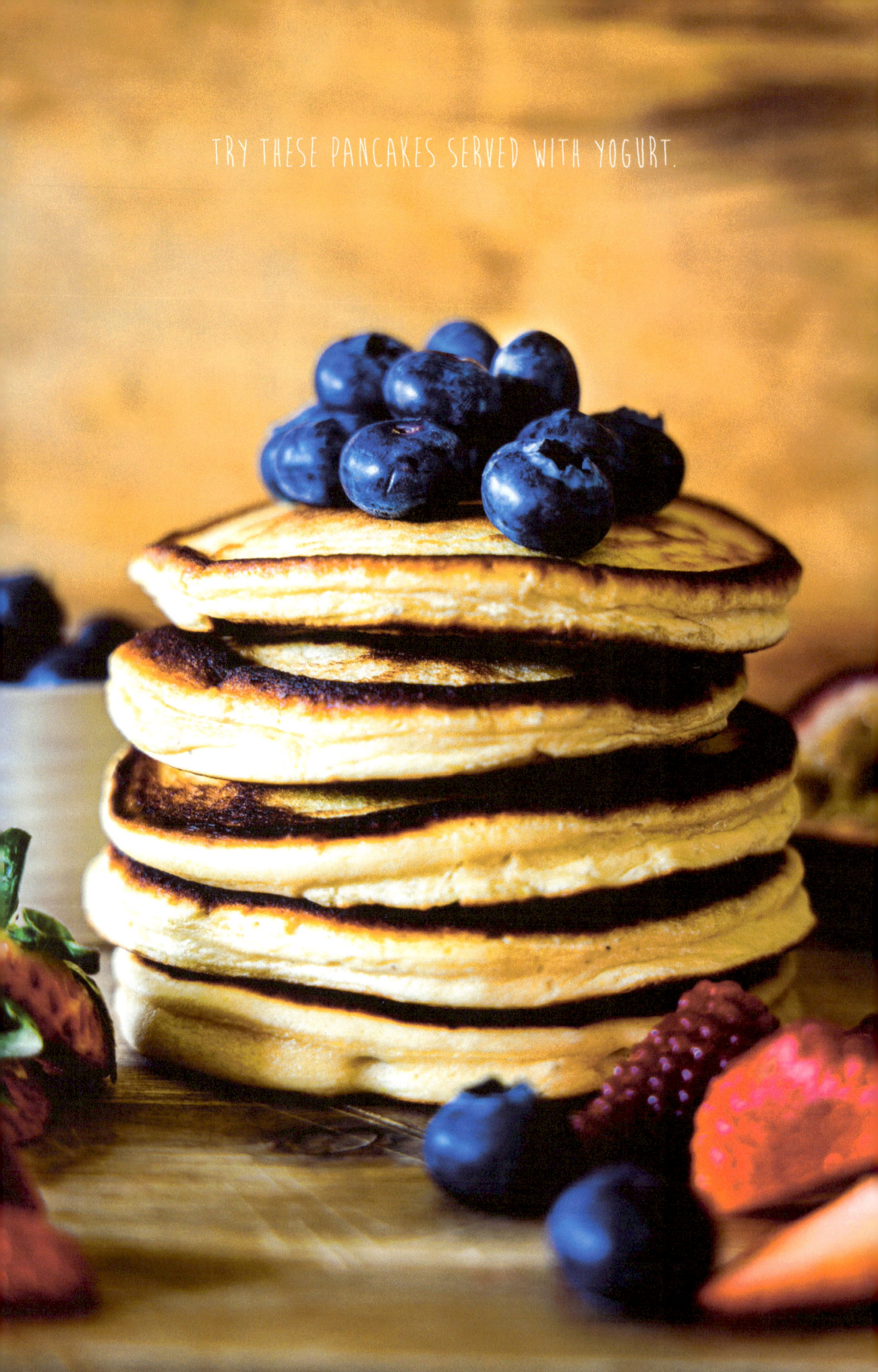

FLUFFY BANANA PANCAKES WITH BERRIES

I have my typical banana & protein pancake recipe (see page 50), but this is a more traditional pancake batter using flour. I don't typically make this version because I prefer oats over flour as my carbohydrate, but it's more suitable when you want to make tall, round pancakes. Flour is produced from wheat and its main nutritional component is carbohydrate. It has a significant amount of fibre and protein as well. Note that the protein is mostly in the form of gluten.

PREP : 5 MINUTES | COOK : 15 MINUTES | SERVES : 3 (6 PANCAKES)

1 cup white flour

1 banana

3 tsp vanilla extract

½ tsp bi carb soda

1 scoop vanilla protein powder

4 eggs

1 tbs olive oil for cooking

½ cup mixed berries

1 passionfruit, chopped

1 tbs honey

Add the flour, banana, vanilla, bi carb soda, protein powder, and eggs to your bullet blender and blend thoroughly.

Heat a bit of olive oil in your pan on low heat. Add only a small amount as required for each pancake.

Pour the batter steadily into the centre of your pan. Pour to your desired size. You will see your pancake increase in size evenly.

Flip your pancakes when you start to see small air bubbles form. This will only take 1 to 2 minutes. The second side will cook in less time than the first.

Serve with berries and passionfruit on top. Drizzle with honey.

Add 1 cup of milk to make the batter go further.

CALORIES 572.6KCAL | PROTEIN 25.3G | CARBS 57.1G | FATS 27G

Protein French Toast with Berries

It's hard to resist French toast at the best of times. Now, it's even more appealing since it's packed with protein and has the sweetness of berries, honey, and a dusting of cinnamon! This recipe is another energy-packed meal you can make in just 15 minutes.

PREP : 5 MINUTES | COOK : 10 MINUTES | SERVES : 2

1 tbs olive oil for cooking

2 eggs

1 scoop whey protein

1 tbs vanilla extract

4 slices sourdough bread

1 cup mixed berries

1 tsp cinnamon

1 tbs honey

Heat the olive oil in your pan with olive oil on medium heat.

Whisk the eggs with the protein powder and vanilla extract in a wide bowl.

Soak both sides of each slice of bread in the egg mixture. Add straight to your pan.

Fry all 4 slices at once for about 5 minutes on each side until the egg is golden and crispy.

Serve the French toast with a scattering of berries. Dust some cinnamon on top and drizzle with a little honey.

CALORIES 478.8KCAL | PROTEIN 34.4G | CARBS 42.1G | FATS 19.2G

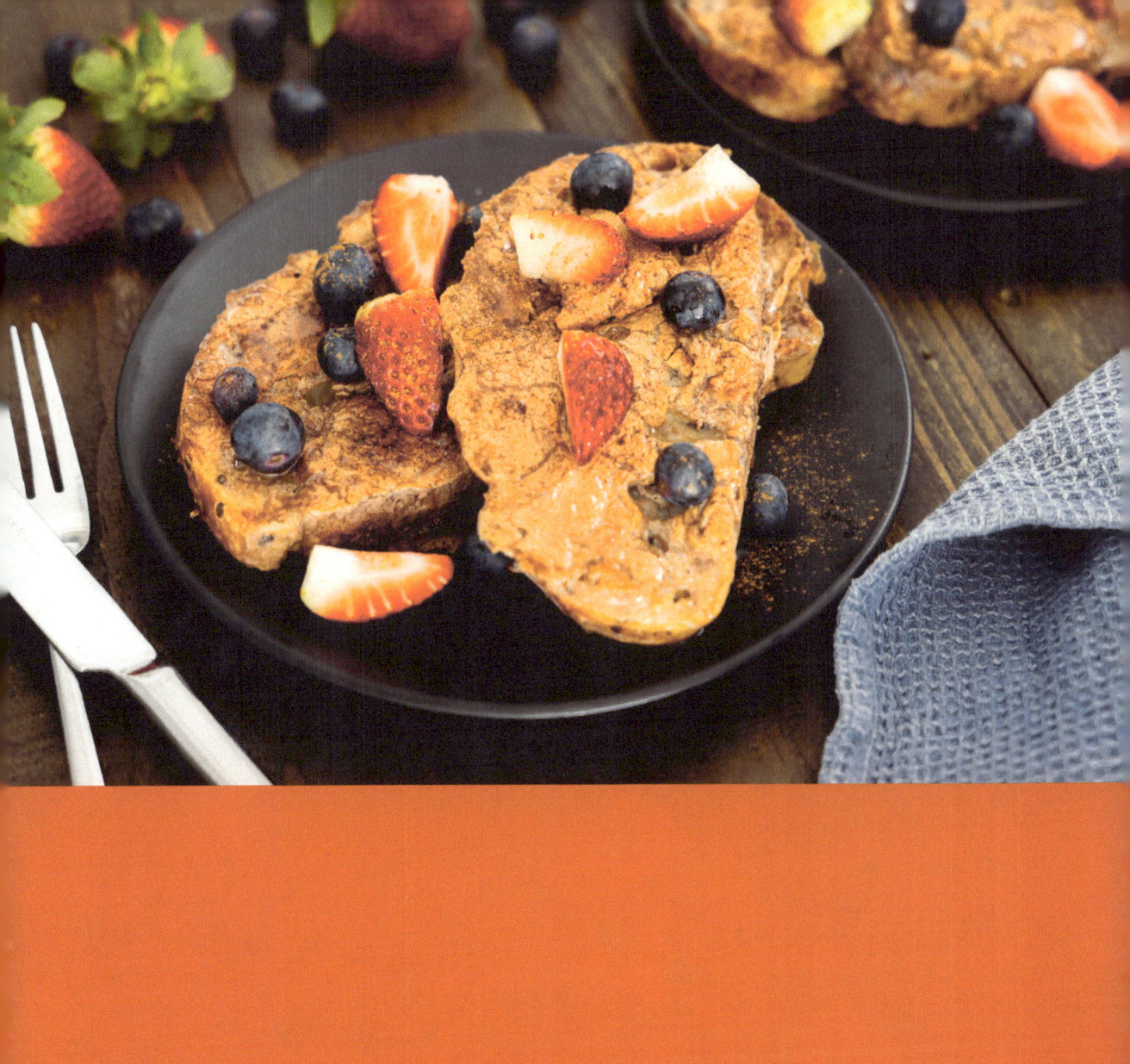

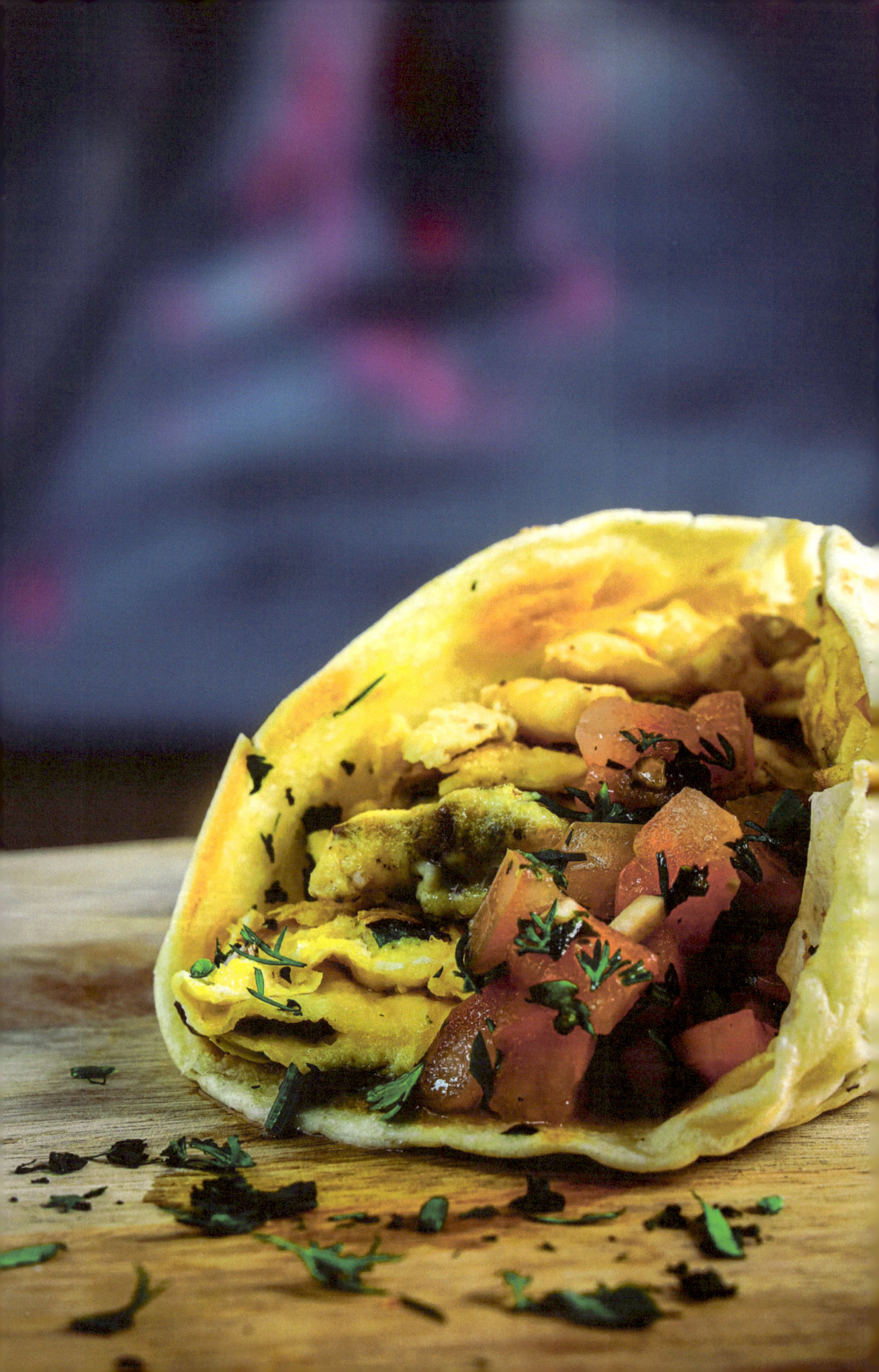

BREAKFAST BURRITO WITH TOMATO SALSA

This is a great way to make fancy eggs. The tomato salsa goes well with scrambled eggs and is a fresh option for breakfast. It's also perfect as a quick snack.

PREP : 10 MINUTES | COOK : 12 MINUTES | SERVES : 1

1 tbs olive oil for cooking

2 soft tortilla wraps

3 mushrooms, finely diced

4 eggs

1 tbs milk

Pinch of salt & pepper

Tomato Salsa

½ tomato, finely diced

Juice of ½ lime

½ tbs olive oil

1 tsp freshly chopped parsley

1 tsp freshly chopped basil

1 tsp freshly chopped dill

Pinch of salt & pepper

Mix together all the salsa ingredients in a bowl. Set aside.

Heat the olive oil in your frying pan on medium heat.

Warm your tortillas in the microwave or fry them in the pan for 2 minutes on each side just to brown them. Set aside on a plate.

Add the mushrooms to the pan for a minute to brown.

Whisk the eggs with splash of milk in a bowl and pour into the pan.

When the eggs start to cook, after about a minute, start folding them with a spatula like an omelette or scramble them with a wooden spoon. They will cook fully in 2 to 3 minutes.

Plate up by adding the eggs and mushrooms to both wraps and topping with the salsa.

Add salt & pepper as desired. Wrap and eat!

CALORIES 745.5KCAL | PROTEIN 36G | CARBS 39G | FATS 49.5G

GREEK COFFEE

There's no doubt that I love my Greek coffee and the connection it gives me to my Greek culture. It has a strong flavour, but there are a few ways to make it: sketo/plain (without sugar), metrio/medium (1:1 coffee:sugar), and glyko/sweet (1:2 coffee:sugar). However you like it, making Greek coffee requires a little technique and attention. Don't ask me why Greek coffee is often made with Turkish coffee...

PREP : 1 MINUTES | COOK : 3 MINUTES | SERVES : 1

1 heaped tsp (7g) Turkish coffee

1 tsp (5g) raw sugar

Water

Other

Briki

Greek coffee cup

(metrio/medium sweetness)

Add the Turkish coffee and raw sugar into your briki.

Fill your cup with tap water to fill the required amount in your briki.

Now, don't mix! The trick to producing the foam (kaimaki) on top is to allow the coffee to mix as it cooks.

Put your briki on low to medium heat for about 2 minutes. The real timing to boiling the coffee is to remove it from the heat at exactly the right moment. Just before the water starts to bubble, remove it from the heat. You will burn the coffee if you allow it to bubble/boil continuously.

Pour into your cup to serve. When serving, pour the foam evenly into each cup before filling them all up.

Because Greek coffee can be quite strong, it is served with a glass of water. Sip it slowly to enjoy the aroma. Don't drink the "mud" that's left in the bottom of your cup.

CALORIES 28.4KCAL | PROTEIN 1.2G | CARBS 5.9G | FATS 0G

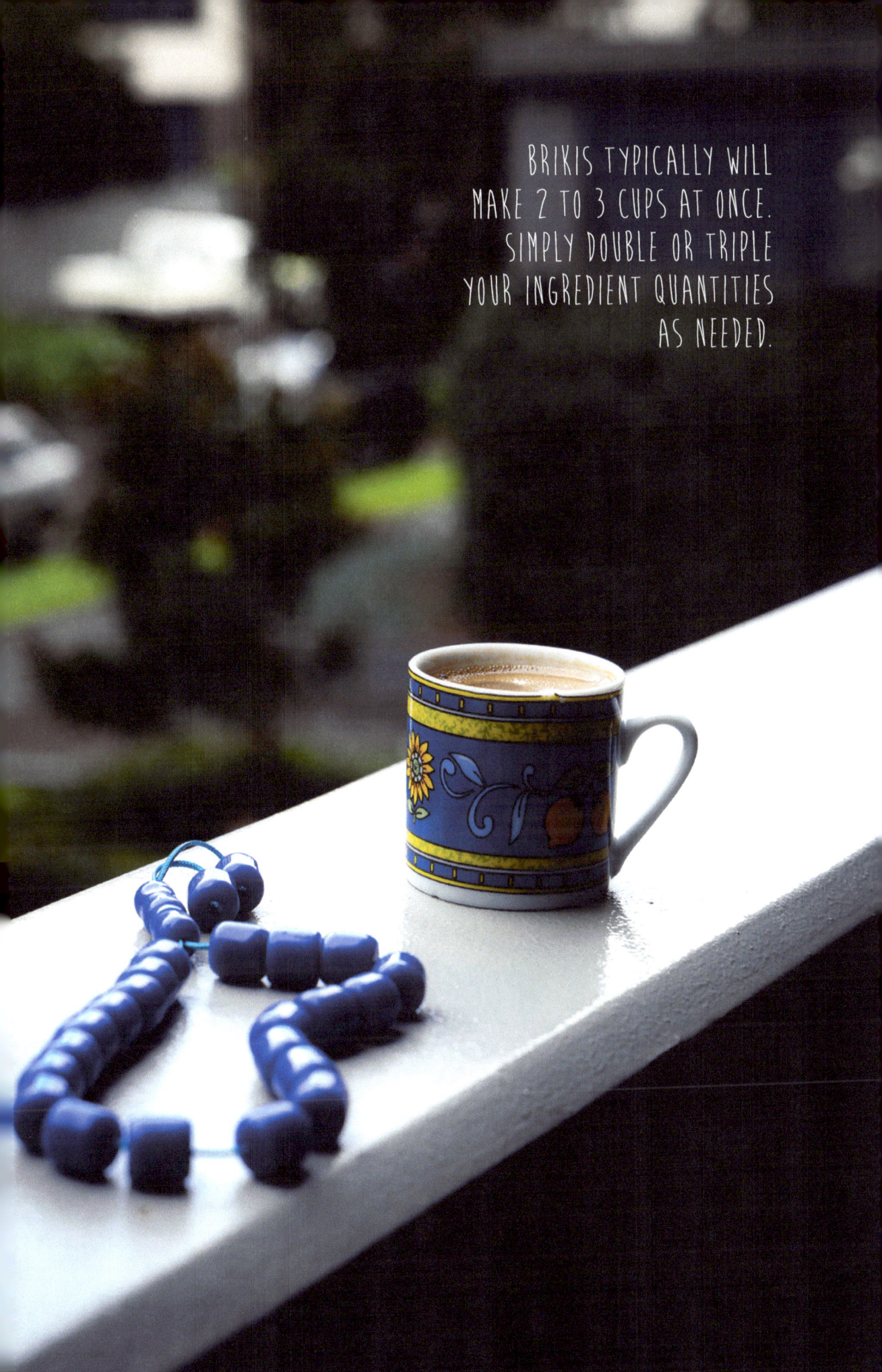

Brikis typically will make 2 to 3 cups at once. Simply double or triple your ingredient quantities as needed.

MEALS

Spaghetti Bolognese with Veggies

If this book is about learning the basics, then study this page twice! This version of spaghetti bolognese is packed with herbs and veggies that really are delightful to the taste buds. So don't fear! Load your Bolognese with veggies for flavour and the added nutritional bonus.

PREP : 10 MINUTES | COOK : 1 HOUR | SERVES : 5

2 tbs olive oil for cooking

3 garlic cloves, finely diced

1kg turkey mince

1 cup finely diced celery

1 carrot, finely diced or grated

1 cup mushrooms, finely diced

⅓ cup mixed freshly chopped basil, parsley & oregano

700g bottle passata

410g can crushed tomatoes

500g pasta (spaghetti)

Heat the olive oil in your frying pan on medium heat. Fry the garlic for 10 seconds before adding your mince.

Cook the mince until it's just brown, about 10 minutes. Use a wooden spoon to continually break the mince apart while turning it over.

Add your diced veggies and herbs. Thoroughly mix with the mince and cook for another minute.

Pour in the bottle of passata and can of crushed tomatoes. Mix thoroughly.

Turn your heat down to low and let simmer for 40 to 60 minutes, stirring every 10 minutes. The passata will reduce to a thicker sauce over this time. Add water if the passata reduces too quickly.

Cook your pasta according to package directions before you're ready to serve. Serve the sauce over the pasta.

Serving includes 1 cup of pasta 14.6g protein; 78.8g carbs; 1.6g fat; 388kcal.

Steam other veggies like broccoli and green beans to serve as a side.

You can substitute the turkey mince with the more traditional option of beef mince.

Add ½ onion (diced) if desired which is traditionally in bolognese too.

CALORIES 680KCAL | PROTEIN 50.6G | CARBS 88.1G | FATS 13.9G

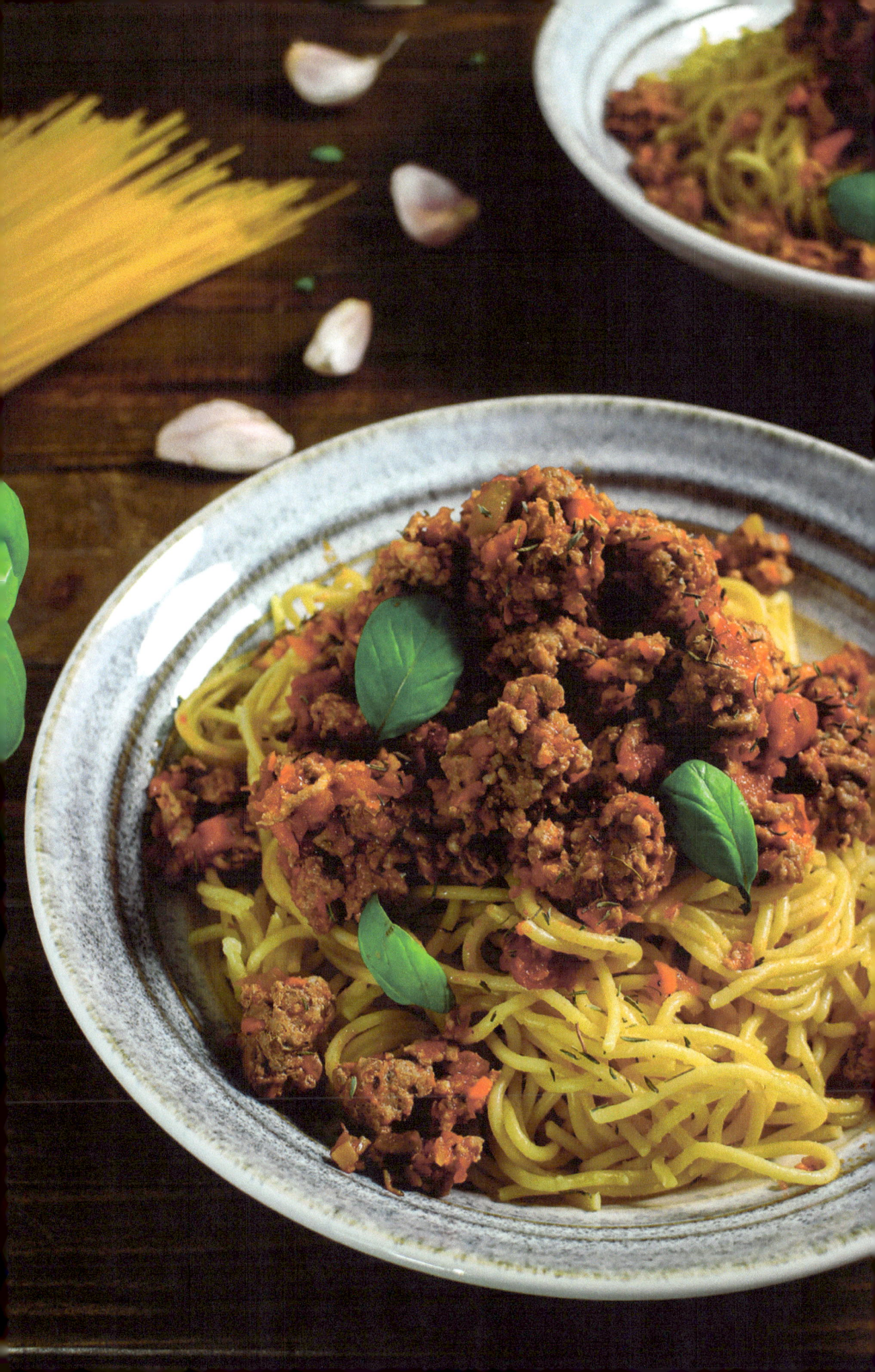

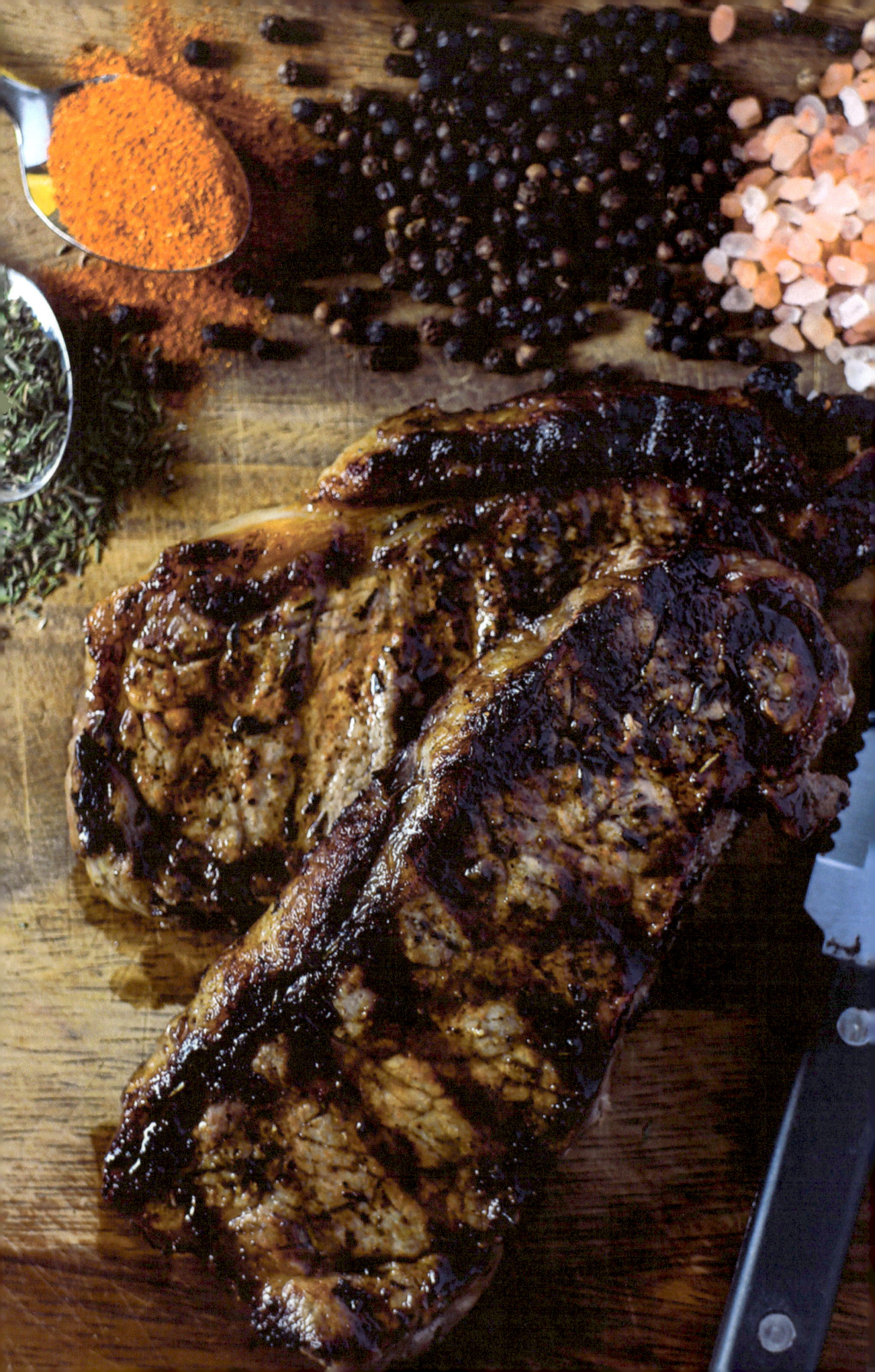

CHARGRILLED STEAK WITH MIXED HERBS

You're sure to impress when you get a steak right! It's soft, juicy, and just charred on the outside. Adding the right marinade to enhance the flavour of the meat will take it from good to great. This is my go-to combination.

PREP : 20 MINUTES | COOK : 20 MINUTES | SERVES : 1

⅓ tsp mixed freshly chopped thyme & oregano

⅓ tsp salt

⅓ tsp pepper

⅓ tsp paprika

1 tbs olive oil, plus more for cooking

Juice of ½ lemon

300g porterhouse steak

Use a mortar & pestle to crush together the herbs and spices.

Add the olive oil and lemon juice and mix.

Pour half of the marinade over each side of your steak. Rub it in evenly.

Let the steak rest for at least 15 minutes at room temperature. This brings the best flavour from the steak.

Heat your BBQ or fry pan to high heat. You want to hear that sizzle when the steak hits the pan. A hot pan will sear the steak and give it a nice crust.

Lay the steak in the pan away from you to avoid hot oil splattering at you. Turn the steak while it's still pink in the middle (watch the side of the steak cook as the colour changes up towards the centre). Baste with some of the marinade after turning.

The steak will continue to cook while at rest, so achieve your perfection on the plate by taking it off the heat early while it's still pink in the centre.

Let the steak rest for 5 minutes before serving. Baste with any leftover marinade for extra flavour.

Marinate your steak ½ day prior to barbequing for the best flavour.

Serving this with 1 cup of baked potatoes and 1 cup of veggies adds 10.7g protein; 36.4g carbs; 10.3g fat; 281.1kcal.

CALORIES 493.5KCAL | PROTEIN 60.6G | CARBS 0.9G | FATS 27.5G

STEAK SANDWICH

Everyone should know how to make a delicious steak sandwich. Making it yourself means you won't compromise with the quality. It's a quick and healthy option in your meal plan.

PREP : 10 MINUTES | COOK : 30 MINUTES | SERVES : 2

200g porterhouse steak or minute steaks

2 eggs

2 thick slices of bread

½ avocado

½ cup leafy greens

½ tomato, sliced

4 slices canned beetroot

Lemon marinade

Pinch each of salt, pepper & oregano

Juice of ½ lemon

1 tbs olive oil

Mix together the marinade ingredients in a bowl large enough to hold the steak.

Marinate your steak for 20 minutes or up to 2 hours.

Preheat your fry pan or barbeque over medium heat.

Cook the steak to medium, flipping once halfway through. Fry your eggs with the steak. They normally cook quickly, so I time it with the second half of the steak.

Finely slice the porterhouse steak or stick with the full minute steak.

Toast the bread.

Build your sandwich: Spread the avocado on the toast, then layer the leafy greens, tomato, beetroot, eggs, and steak on top.

Add sliced cucumber and/or capsicum if desired.

CALORIES 565.8KCAL | PROTEIN 41.5G | CARBS 30.2G | FATS 31G

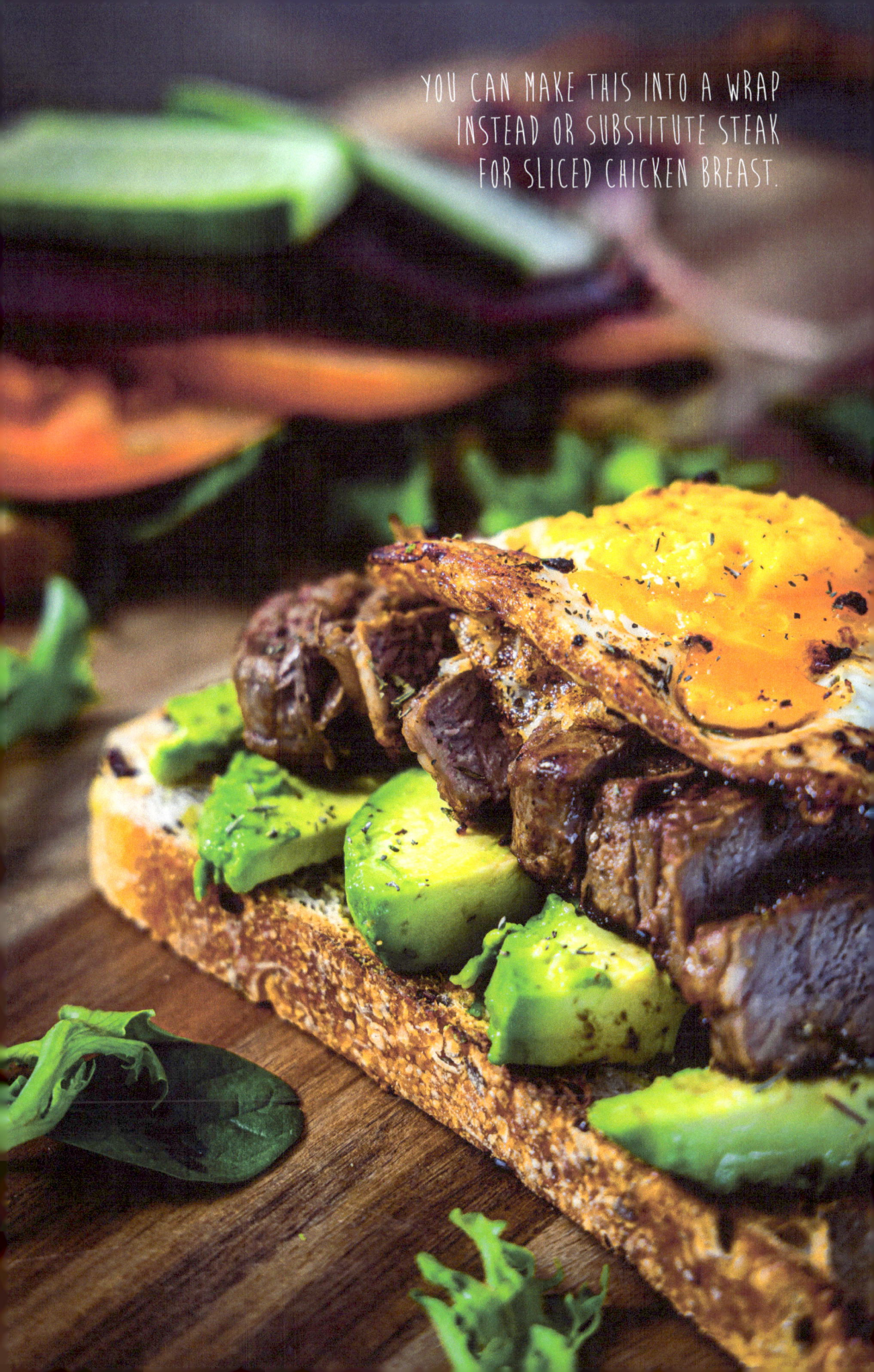

YOU CAN MAKE THIS INTO A WRAP INSTEAD OR SUBSTITUTE STEAK FOR SLICED CHICKEN BREAST.

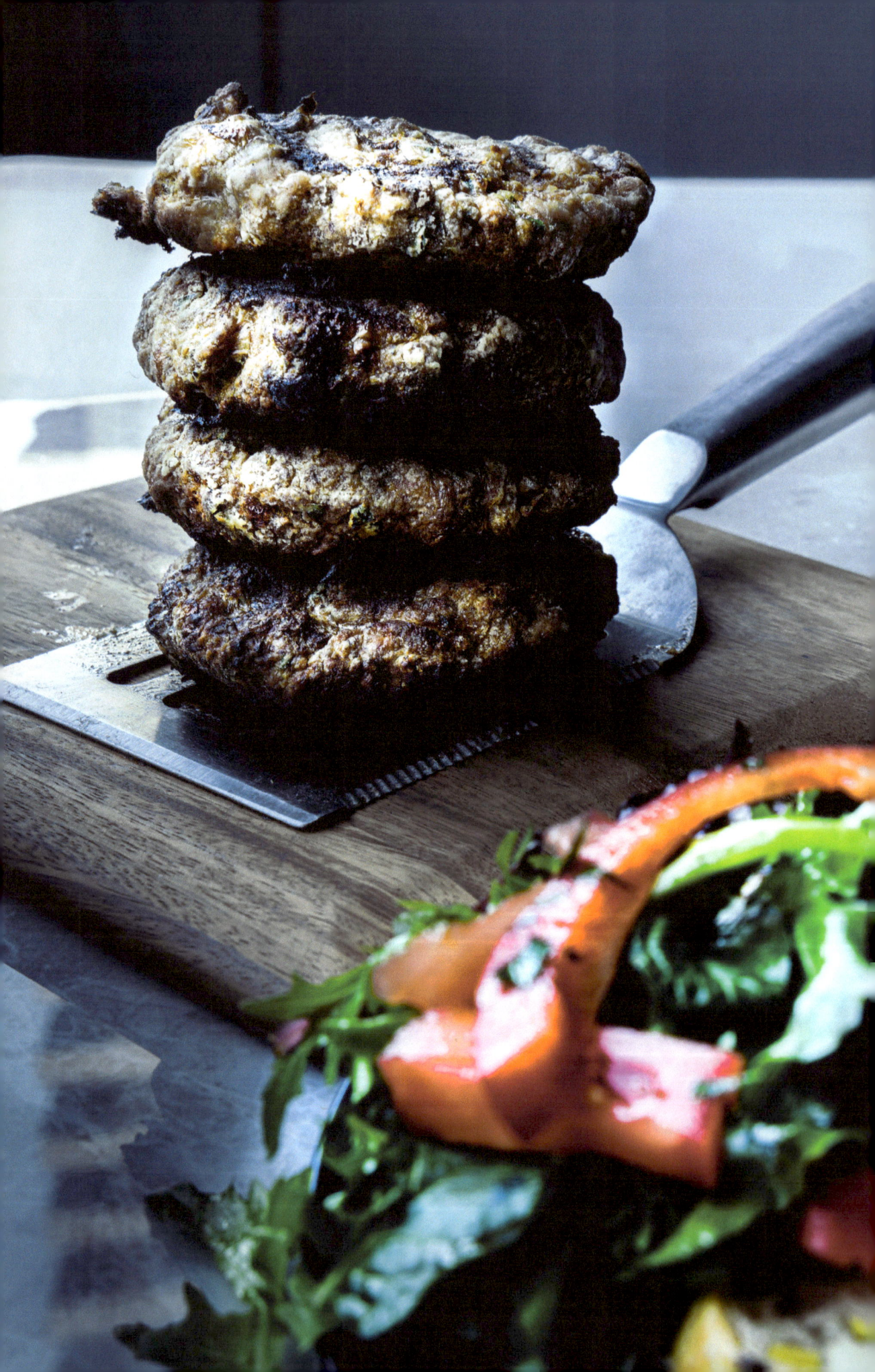

MEATBALLS

Meatballs and burger patties are really one and the same. Yes, you can buy pre-made patties (which I sometimes do because they're quick and the right brands are healthy), but when you really need to pull out all the stops for a tasty and towering burger or spaghetti and meatballs, pull this recipe out of your pocket.

PREP : 50 MINUTES | COOK : 15 MINUTES | SERVES : 6

1kg turkey mince (turkey mince is lowest in fat but beef mince is the traditional choice)

2 eggs

½ cup breadcrumbs

1 tsp mixed salt & pepper

1 small chilli, finely chopped

1 tsp paprika

½ cup freshly chopped parsley

1 cup flour for coating

In a large bowl, mix together all the ingredients (except the flour) thoroughly by hand.

Form your meatballs or patties by taking a handful of mince and rolling it between your hands. Compress it slightly to give it shape and help the mixture stick together. The size and thickness is up to you.

For a crispy texture, roll the meatballs in a tray of flour to lightly coat them.

Stick your meatballs in the fridge for at least 30 minutes before frying.

Cook your meatballs in a frying pan with olive oil over a medium heat. Turn once when you see the patty begin to brown up the side to the centre.

Serve meatballs in spaghetti, a subway sandwich, or flatten into patties for hamburgers.

Serving these with two slices of sourdough toast to make burgers adds 12.4g protein; 23.5g carbs; 5.9g fat; 196.7kcal.

CALORIES 456.1KCAL | PROTEIN 41.9G | CARBS 37.7G | FATS 15.3G

CHICKEN BREAST WITH LEMON & OREGANO MARINADE

This seasoning is my go-to when cooking chicken breasts, whether baking in the oven or barbequing. The best flavour is on a charcoal barbeque because you can baste the chicken while it's on the grill and the smoke adds to the overall flavour. If you throw it in the oven, just season and baste when serving.

PREP : 15 MINUTES | COOK : 15 MINUTES | SERVES : 4

1 kg chicken breast

Seasoning

½ tsp salt

½ tsp pepper

1 tsp vegeta gourmet stock powder

2 tsp oregano

Juice of ½ lemon

1 tbs olive oil

Marinade

½ tsp salt

½ tsp pepper

Juice of 1 lemon

1 tsp oregano

1 tbs olive oil

Prepare the chicken breast by cutting it into smaller fillets to help it cook evenly. Cut off the tenderloin and cut the breast in half through the middle.

Use a mortar & pestle to crush the salt, pepper, vegeta gourmet stock powder, and oregano. Sprinkle the spices evenly over the chicken, coating both sides.

Drizzle the juice from ½ lemon and 1 tbs olive oil over the chicken.

Toss the chicken pieces together to get an even coating.

Prepare the lemon marinade by mixing all the ingredients together in a separate bowl. Keep to the side when barbequing and serving.

To cook in the oven: Preheat your oven to 180°C and set it to grill mode. Throw the chicken in an oven tray under the grill for 15 minutes. It should have a slightly crispy top.

To cook on the BBQ: Preheat your barbeque on medium heat. Put the chicken on and turn once when the bottom is golden. Grill for 5 to 10 minutes per side depending on your heat. Watch for flame flare-ups if the oil drips. When you turn the chicken, baste the top side with your marinade. Save the rest of the marinade for serving.

Drizzle the spare marinade on the chicken when serving.

If you want this as a low-calorie option, use only enough olive oil for cooking. Chicken packs 55.8g protein, 4g fat and just 259.2kcal per 250g serving.

CALORIES 324.9KCAL | PROTEIN 56G | CARBS 0.9G | FATS 10.9G

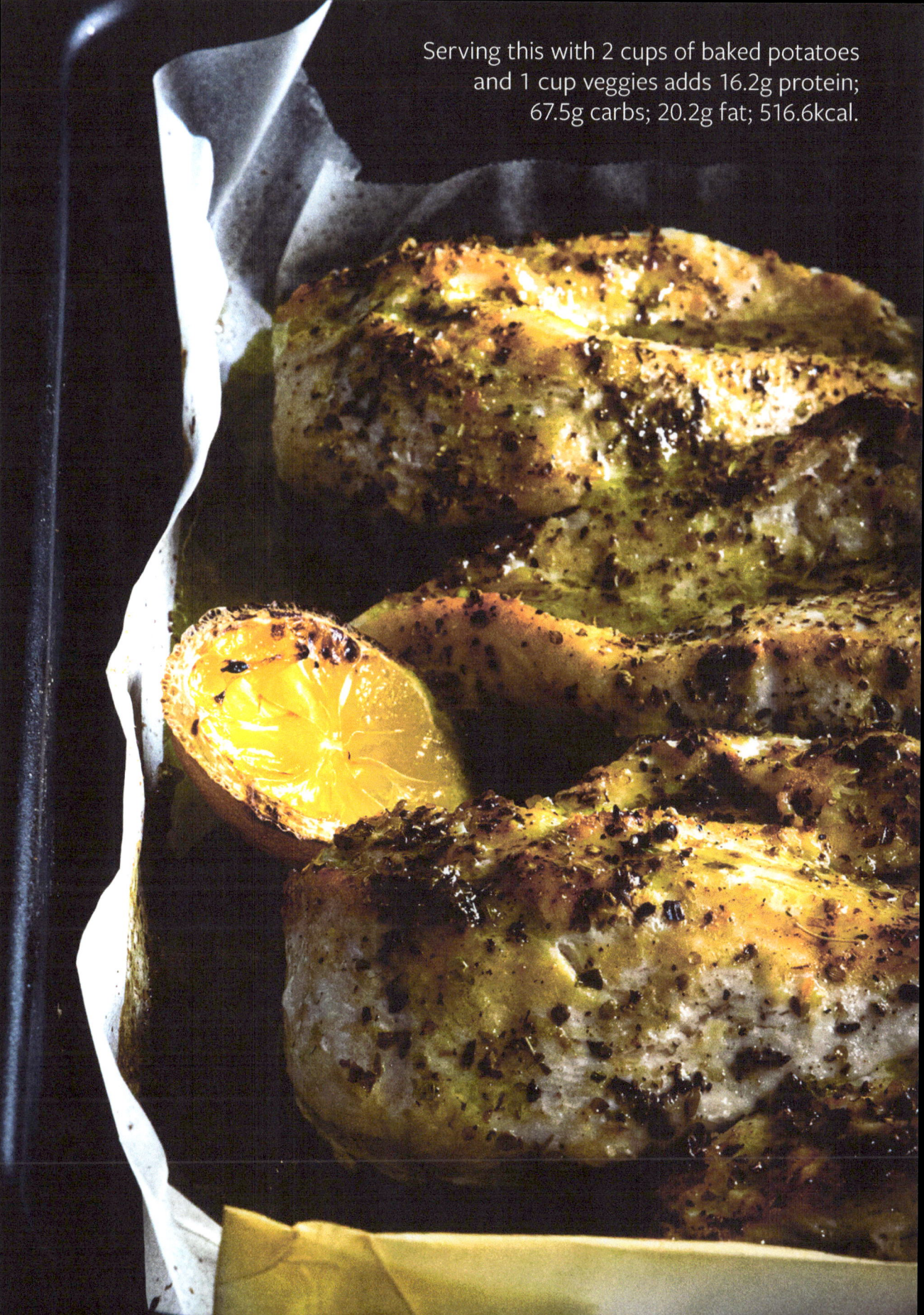

Serving this with 2 cups of baked potatoes and 1 cup veggies adds 16.2g protein; 67.5g carbs; 20.2g fat; 516.6kcal.

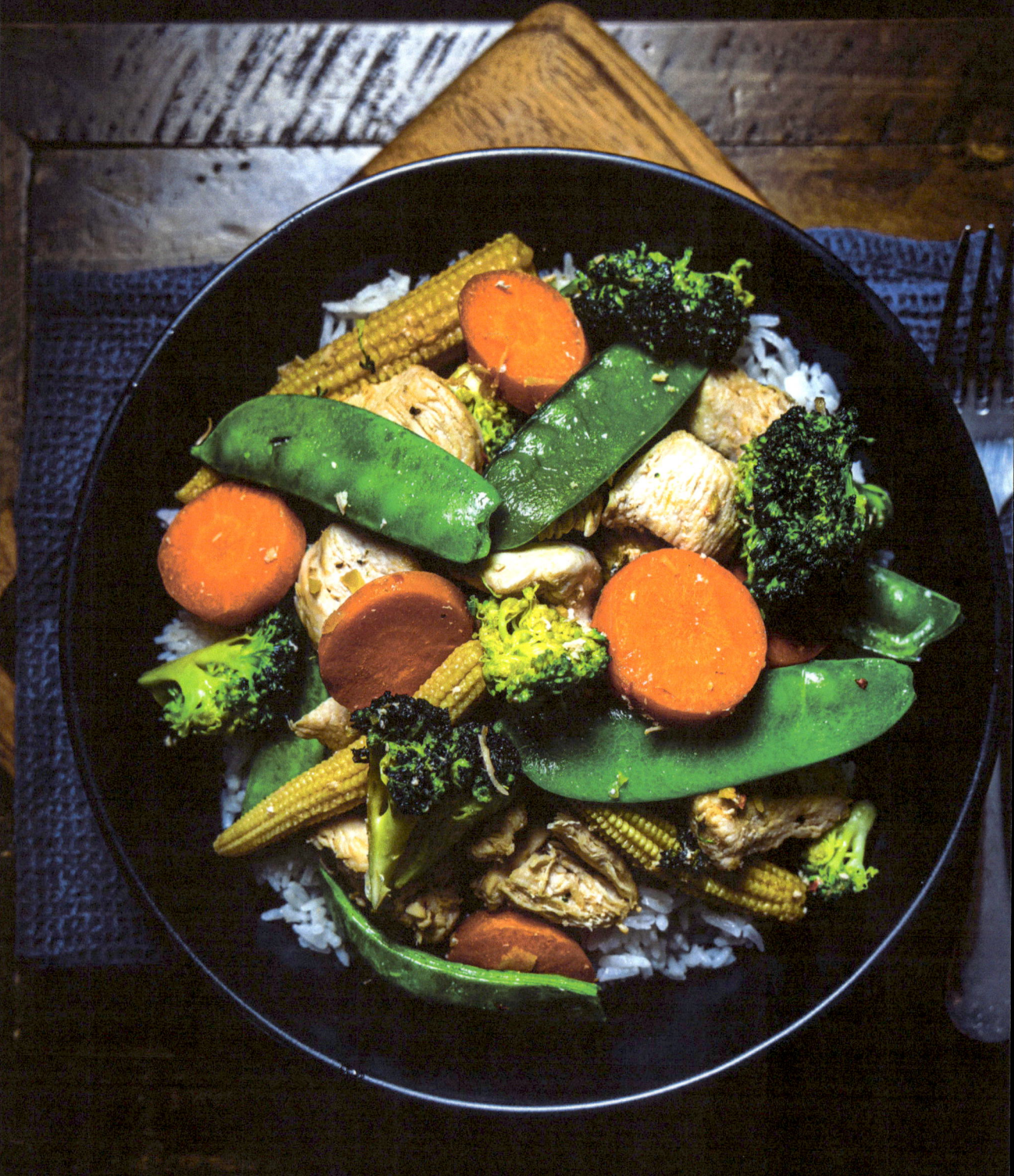

A STIR-FRY IS YOUR OPPORTUNITY FOR VARIETY AND EXPERIMENTATION. TRY ADDING GREEN BEANS, MUSHROOMS, AND SESAME SEEDS.

CHICKEN STIR-FRY WITH VEGGIES & HERBS

What is the second word in stir-fry? FRY! Now is the time to cook on high heat. Use peanut oil which heats up smoking hot without burning, keeping your veggies crunchy and your chicken crisp. Don't make my rookie mistake of using medium heat because it will all stew together and taste terrible. A stir-fry can be your go-to meal for getting more veggies into your meal plan.

PREP : 15 MINUTES | COOK : 10 MINUTES | SERVES : 5

1 kg chicken breasts

2 tbs peanut oil for cooking

1 cup chopped broccoli

1 carrot, chopped

1 cup chopped snow peas

½ cup corn

Marinade

1 tsp minced fresh ginger

1 garlic clove, chopped

4 tbs soy sauce

2 tbs sesame oil

2 tbs honey

⅓ cup mixed freshly chopped parsley & basil

Prepare your chicken by cutting it into bite-size pieces.

Prepare the marinade by mixing together all the ingredients.

Heat up your pan or wok on high heat and add the peanut oil.

Flash-fry your chicken for about 5 minutes until cooked through. Leave it on the heat. It will brown with the veggies.

Add the broccoli and carrot first as those take the longest to cook. At the same time, add the marinade and mix thoroughly. Continue stirring every few seconds for 3 to 4 minutes.

In the last minute, throw in the snow peas and corn. The snow peas only need a minute and will retain their crunch.

Remove from the heat and serve.

Using a wok, if you have one, has advantages but they need a powerful gas stove. Woks are better for cooking on high heat because the heat transfers up the sides, creating a larger cooking surface.

Serving this with 1 cup of white rice adds 4.3g protein; 57.6g carbs; 0.2g fat; 249.4kcal.

CALORIES 340.4KCAL | PROTEIN 47.9G | CARBS 12.9G | FATS 10.8G

Chicken Schnitzel with Herbs & Lemon Zest

Schnitzel is a crowd favourite and a safe bet to satisfy your dinner party. The beauty of making the schnitzel yourself is that you can infuse the breadcrumbs with the flavours you really want.

PREP : 20 MINUTES | COOK : 30 MINUTES | SERVES : 5

- 1kg chicken breasts
- 300g breadcrumbs
- ½ tsp mixed salt & pepper
- 1 tsp paprika
- Zest & juice of 1 lemon
- ¼ cup freshly chopped parsley
- ¼ cup freshly chopped basil
- 1 cup plain flour
- 3 eggs
- Olive oil as needed for cooking

Cut the chicken breasts down the middle and flatten them for cooking.

Pat the chicken dry with paper towel. It helps them get crispy while cooking.

Pour the breadcrumbs into a large bowl. Add the salt, pepper, paprika, lemon zest, parsley, and basil to the breadcrumbs. Mix thoroughly.

Add the flour to a second bowl and whisk the eggs in a third bowl.

Lay the chicken in the flour. Coat both sides and the edges.

Move the chicken into the egg bowl. Again, coat both sides.

Finally, lay the chicken in the breadcrumbs. Grab the crumbs and compact it into the chicken on both sides and the edges.

Preheat a frying pan over medium heat with a thin layer of olive oil. The schnitzel will crisp up when cooked as a mini deep fry.

Fry for 5 minutes on each side. Repeat with the additional schnitzels, adding more olive oil to the pan with each batch.

Squeeze the lemon over the top and serve.

> Schnitzel is a relatively high-calorie meal on its own. Serving this meal with veggies, like any meal, helps you feel full without going over your required calorie intake. Veggies are free calories.

CALORIES 645.7KCAL | PROTEIN 51.1G | CARBS 58.8G | FATS 22.9G

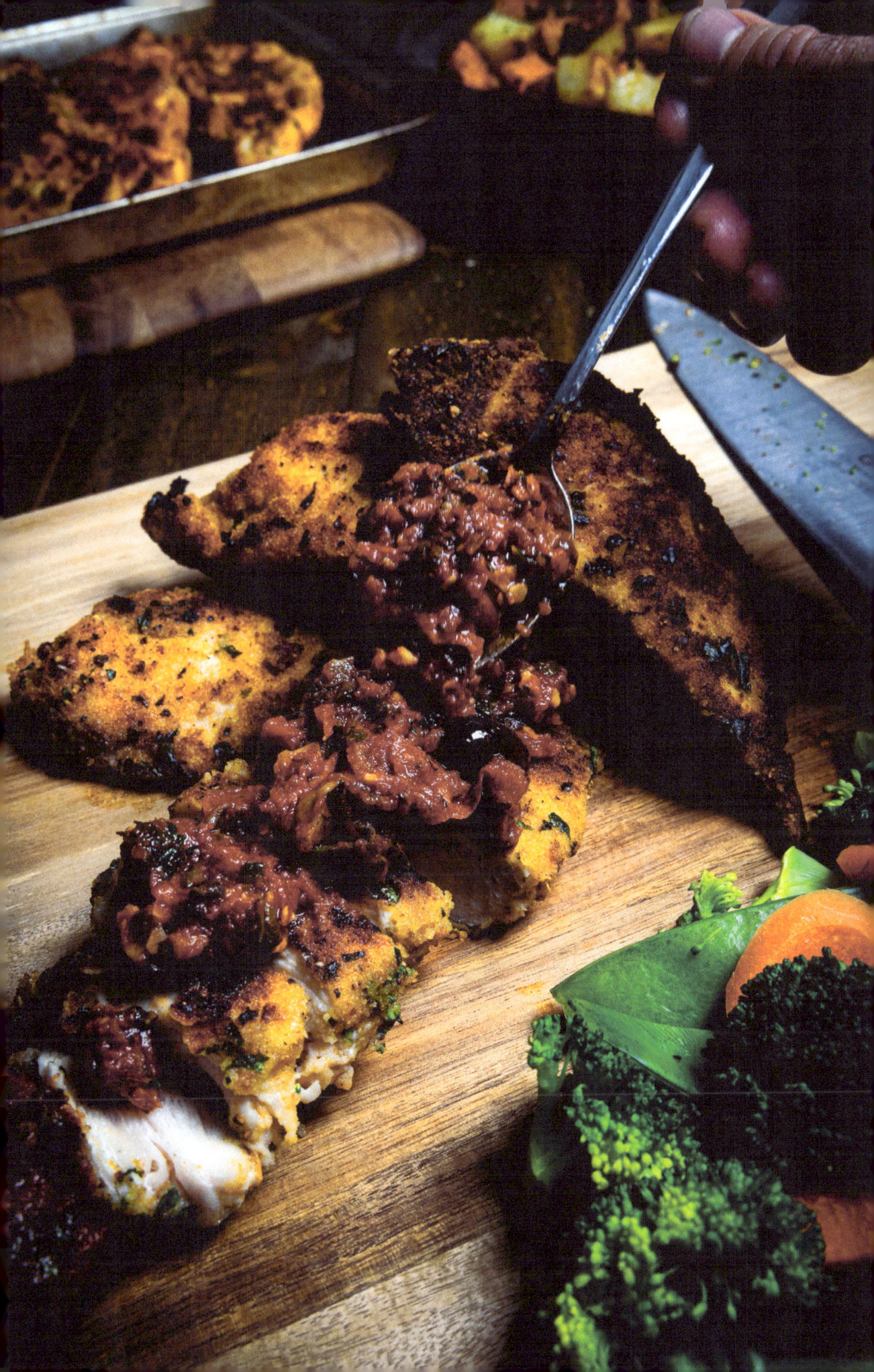

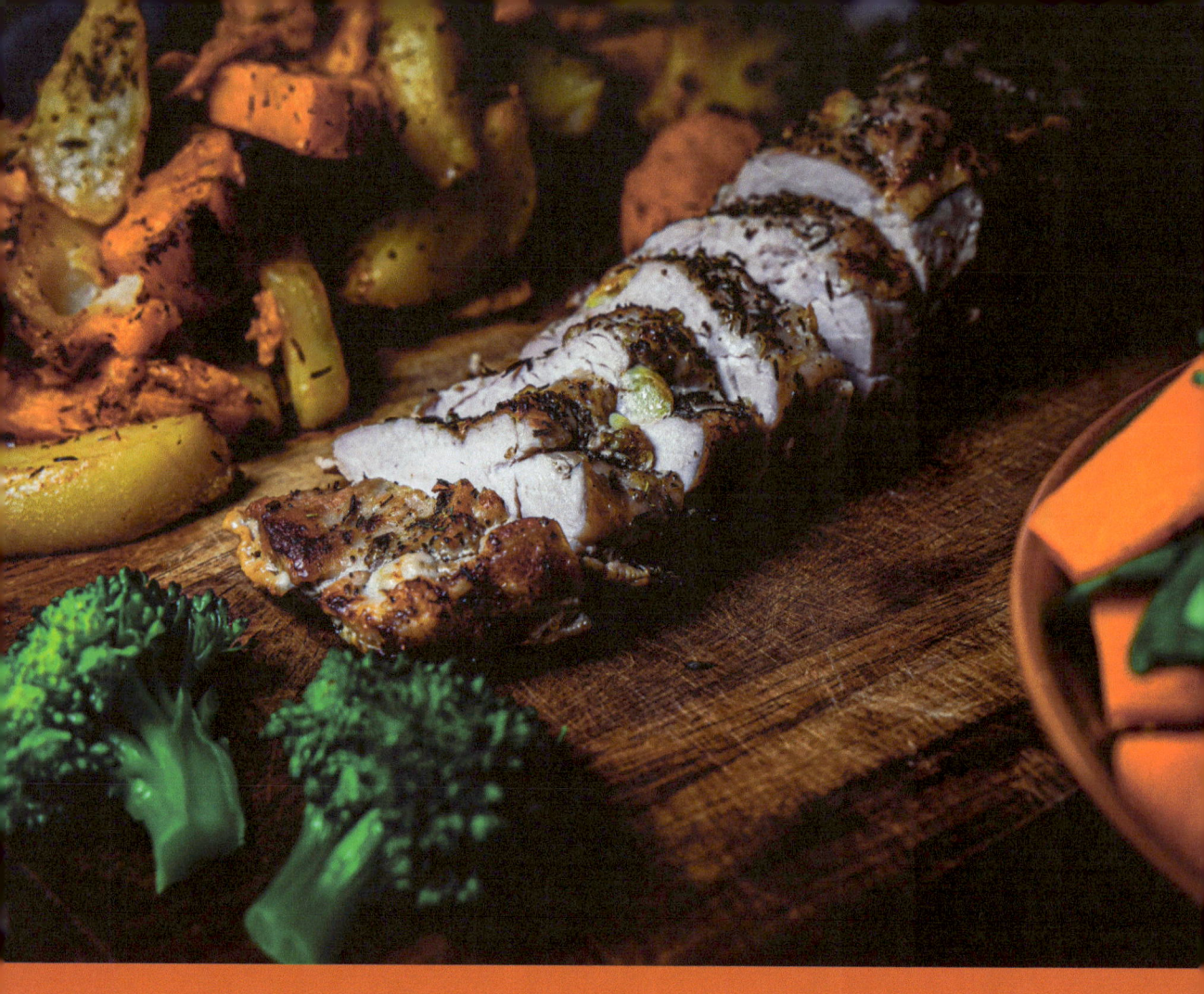

Cooking this cut of meat in the oven is easiest because it cooks through, plus the heat from the grill crisps the top for a nice texture.

PORK LOIN WITH GARLIC AND LEMON

I love this cut because the meat is super tender and a clean source of protein. It's well priced too and easy to cook in the oven. Dress it with any of your favourite healthy sauces; my favourite is simply garlic and lemon.

PREP : 5 MINUTES | COOK : 20 MINUTES | SERVES : 2

450g pork loin

⅓ tsp rosemary

⅓ tsp salt

⅓ tsp pepper

½ garlic clove, finely chopped

Juice of ½ lemon

1 tbs olive oil

Preheat your oven on grill mode to 180°C.

Place the pork in an oven tray. Cut about 10 slits into the pork with the tip of your knife.

Season the pork well by rubbing in the rosemary, salt, and pepper on all sides.

Push the garlic into the slits.

Drizzle with some of the lemon juice and the olive oil.

Place under the grill for 20 minutes, until the top is crispy.

Serve with another squeeze of lemon juice.

Serving this with 1 cup of baked potatoes and 1 cup of veggies adds 10.7g protein; 36.4g carbs; 10.3g fat; 281.1kcal.

CALORIES 314.1G | PROTEIN 54.4G | CARBS 0.5G | FATS 10.5G

CHILLI & GARLIC PASTA

It's not often you consider frying your pasta. This is a great recipe to give variety to plain, boiled pasta. By frying the pasta you can add so much flavour without it always being in a sauce, and it only takes a couple of extra minutes. Look, act, and feel like a pro with this one!

PREP : 10 MINUTES | COOK : 30 MINUTES | SERVES : 5

1 pack of spaghetti

2 small chillis, finely diced

3 garlic cloves, finely diced

½ cup mushrooms, finely diced

⅓ cup mixed freshly chopped parsley & basil

5–10 tbs olive oil

Bring a pot of water to boil. The trick to cooking pasta and preventing it from sticking together is to add it to rapidly boiling water and stirring immediately to separate the strands.

Add the pasta without breaking it into smaller pieces. Add it to the boiling water vertically. In seconds, the bottom half that's in the water will soften and the pasta will fall into the water further. Use tongs to turn it in the water. Keep turning the pasta in the same direction to separate the strands.

Cook for 5 to 10 minutes. The pasta should still have some bite to it. Drain and set aside.

Divide the chilli, garlic, mushrooms, and herbs into five servings.

Heat 1 to 2 tbs olive oil in your frying pan on medium heat.

Cook each serving separately. So, add a portion of garlic and chilli first to the pan for 20 seconds. Then throw in a portion of pasta. Add additional olive oil with each serving to coat the pasta and help it fry.

Add the herbs and mushrooms. Start turning your pasta to thoroughly mix all of your ingredients. Fry until the pasta is crisp and brown, about 2 minutes, turning every 10 to 20 seconds.

Serve hot.

Serving this with 200g of prawns for additional protein adds 41g protein; 0g carbs; 1.2g fat; 174.8kcal.

CALORIES 640.2KCAL | PROTEIN 15G | CARBS 79.8G | FATS 29G

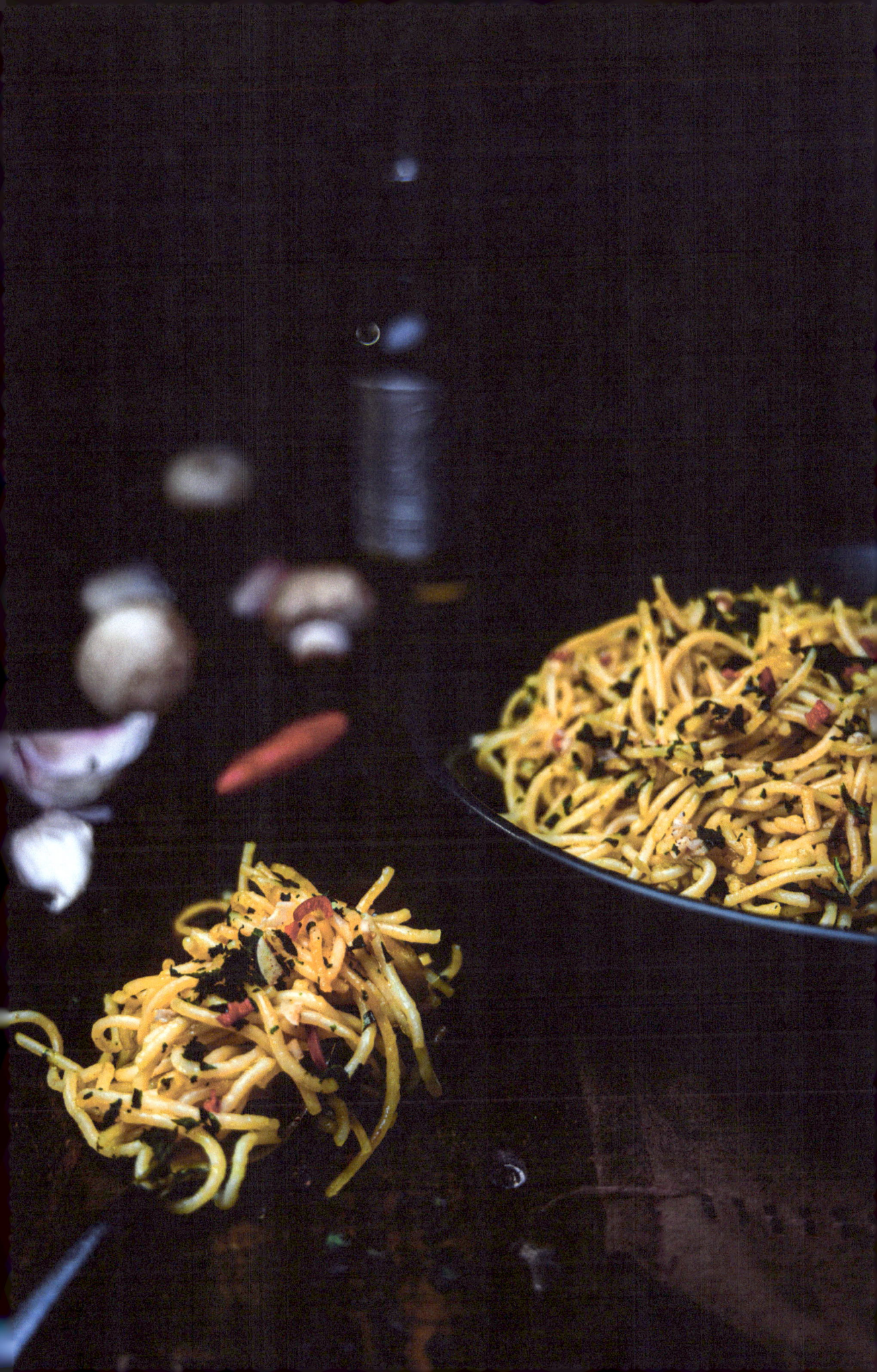

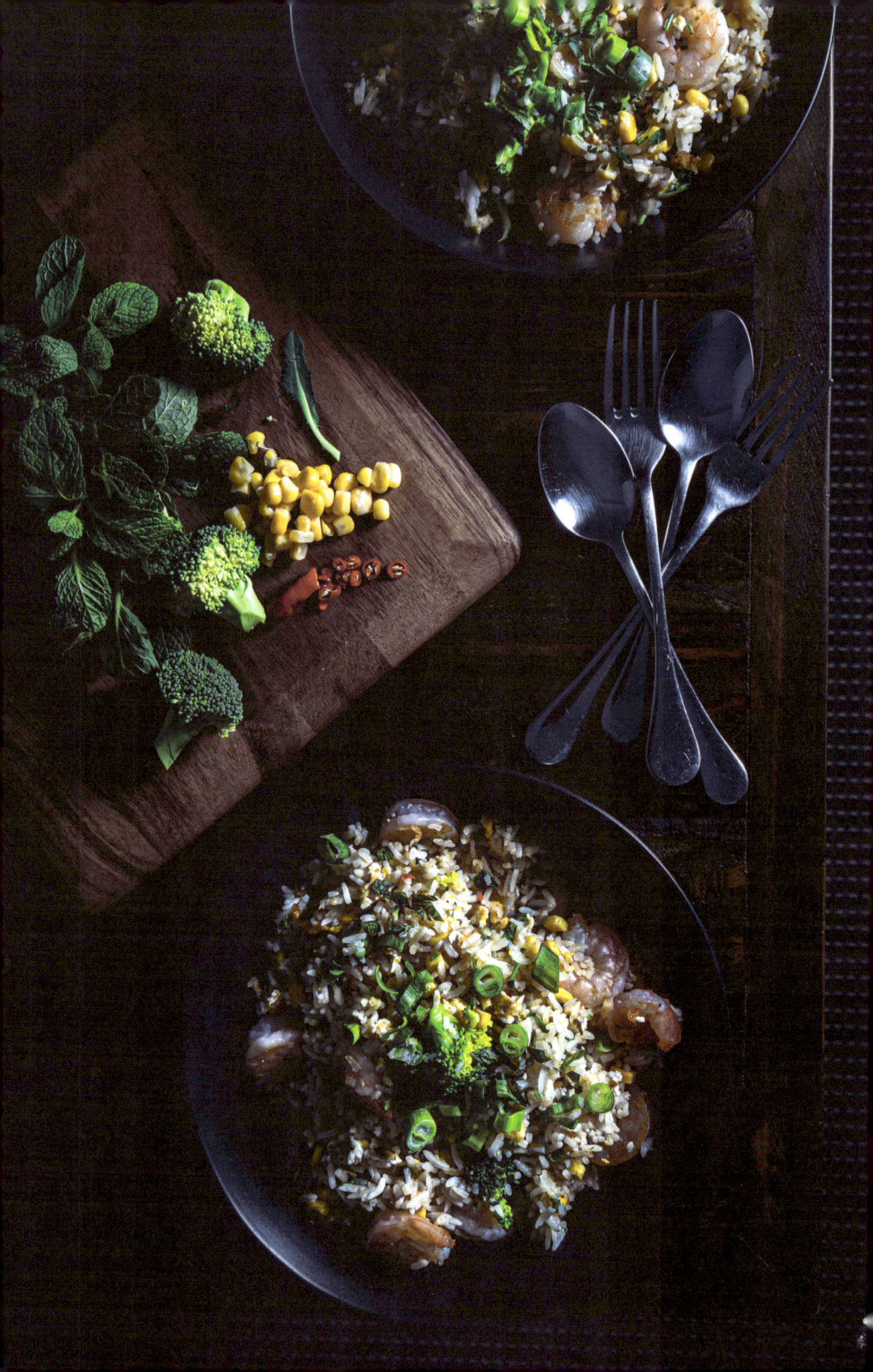

Fried Rice with Prawns

Fried rice is one of those all-in-one dishes that you can throw anything into. The key step is using leftover rice from the night before. You can make this a complete one-pan meal by adding extra veggies like carrots or broccoli.

PREP : 10 MINUTES | COOK : 10 MINUTES | SERVES : 3

3 eggs	Whisk the eggs in a bowl. Set aside.
1 cup bite-size broccoli pieces	Microwave the broccoli in a bowl of water for 3 minutes.
1tbs olive oil for cooking	Heat the olive oil in the pan on medium heat. Fry your prawns for a few minutes until cooked and remove from the pan. Set aside.
300g prawns	
1 small chilli, finely chopped	Add the chilli and ginger to the pan and quickly fry for 30 seconds.
1 tbs finely chopped fresh ginger	
3 cups cooked white rice	Add the eggs and scramble.
⅓ cup mixed freshly chopped parsley, mint & shallots	Add the rice, herbs, corn, prawns, and broccoli, followed by the soy sauce and sesame oil. Stir thoroughly until evenly mixed.
⅓ cup corn	Cook for 2 to 3 minutes, mixing regularly.
1 tbs soy sauce	Turn off the heat. The rice is ready to serve.
1 tbs sesame oil	

> Remember, veggies are free calories, meaning you can eat as much as you like. They are high-fibre carbohydrates so you stay full for longer, plus you get all of the anti-inflammatory benefits for general health.

CALORIES 569.7KCAL | PROTEIN 34.6G | CARBS 59.9G | FATS 21.3G

Spaghetti Marinara

Spaghetti marinara is a calorie-dense meal full of energy potential. I enjoy this meal for the flavour of a homemade marinara sauce with fresh tomatoes, olive oil, and herbs that cannot be matched from a bottle. Cook the spaghetti, seafood, and sauce separately and then bring it together in one pan for a few minutes before serving. I recommend buying seafood marinara mix. You can add bigger prawns and mussels yourself.

PREP : 5 MINUTES | COOK : 30 MINUTES | SERVES : 3

750g seafood marinara mix

1 pack spaghetti

Marinara Sauce

410g can crushed tomatoes

3 tbs olive oil

3 garlic cloves, finely chopped

1 small chilli, finely chopped

1 tbs freshly chopped parsley

1 tbs freshly chopped basil

Pinch of salt & pepper

Coat your pan with peanut oil and preheat on medium-high heat. Bring water to a boil in another pot for your pasta.

Fry your marina mix first in two lots (~375g each). Avoid cooling the pan by adding too much seafood at once (this would cause it to stew). Fry both batches and remove from the heat. Set aside.

Cook your pasta to al dente. It will cook more when you add it to the marinara sauce in a moment. Reserve ½ cup of the pasta water.

Make your marina sauce in the same pan as the seafood. On medium heat, fry the garlic and chilli for 1 minute in olive oil. Pour in the can of crushed tomatoes and simmer with the herbs for another 5 minutes. Transfer the sauce to another bowl for now.

Mix the seafood with the sauce in your portion sizes, i.e. add 250g seafood to your pan with a third of the sauce and roughly 1 cup of pasta.

Add a splash of the pasta water you reserved. Toss the pasta and seafood well on medium heat. Simmer for 2 minutes.

The sauce will start to emulsify and thicken. The starch in the water will help the sauce stick to the pasta evenly and not leave you with a watery sauce.

Take off the heat and serve.

Sprinkle chopped parsley over each serving.

CALORIES 683 KCAL | PROTEIN 44.4G | CARBS 84.6G | FATS 18.6G

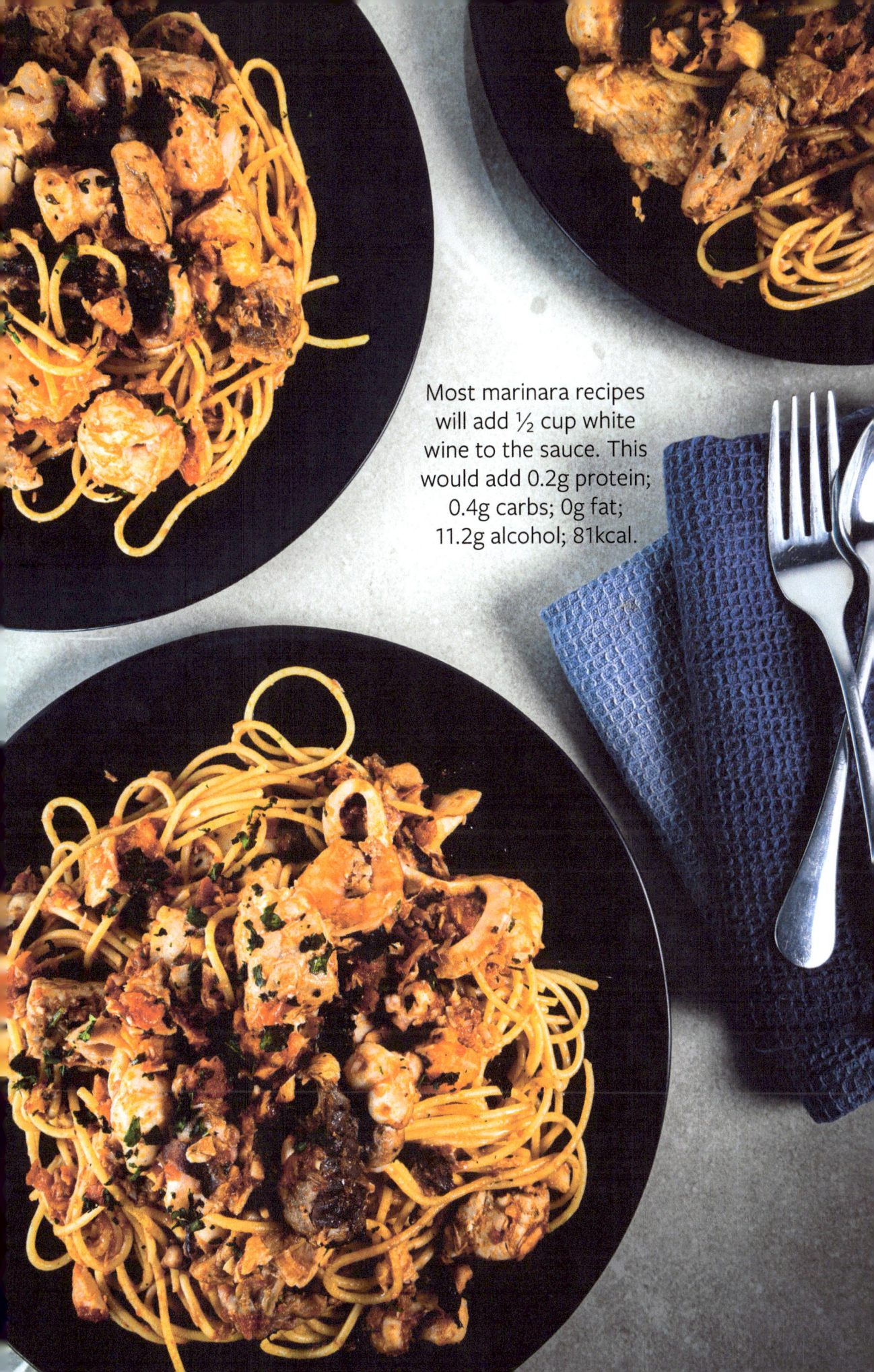

Most marinara recipes will add ½ cup white wine to the sauce. This would add 0.2g protein; 0.4g carbs; 0g fat; 11.2g alcohol; 81kcal.

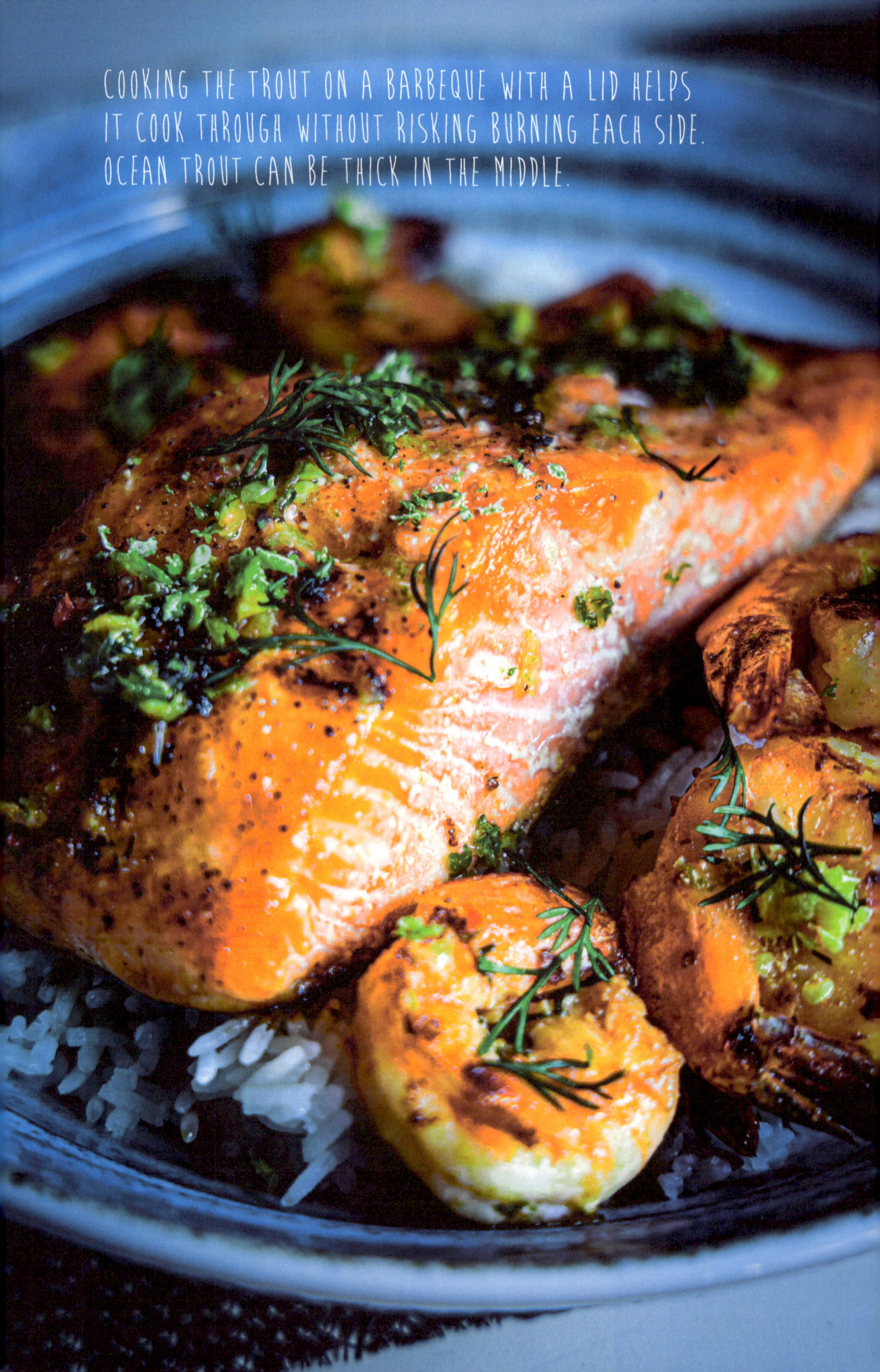

Cooking the trout on a barbeque with a lid helps it cook through without risking burning each side. Ocean trout can be thick in the middle.

OCEAN TROUT & PRAWNS WITH CHIMICHURRI

This is easily one of my favourite recipes in the book. Ocean trout looks like salmon but has a less fishy taste. If you're like me, you will prefer it over salmon from now on. Combined with the flavour of the chimichurri, every bite is mouth-watering. Don't be overwhelmed with this one; it's worth the preparation.

PREP : 2 HOURS | COOK : 20 MINUTES | SERVES : 2

400g ocean trout

200g raw prawn meat

Chimichurri

2 limes

2 tbs olive oil

1 tsp honey

1 tbs soy sauce

1 tsp finely diced ginger

1 small chilli, finely diced

1 tbs freshly chopped dill

Prepare the chimichurri first. Grate the zest from the two limes, then squeeze the juice from both limes into a bowl. Add the olive oil, honey, and soy.

Mix in the ginger, chili, and dill to make the chimichurri.

The fish and prawns come in separate plastic bags. Marinate both by adding ⅓ of the chimichurri into each bag. Coat the seafood by massaging it with your hands. Save the last ⅓ of the chimichurri to dress your fish and prawns when serving.

Let the trout and prawns rest in the fridge for an hour or two or until you prepare the rest of the meal.

Preheat a frying pan or barbeque to medium heat with some olive oil. Start cooking the trout first since it's thicker. Just before the trout browns at the centre, turn it over. It will take roughly 10 minutes on each side depending on the thickness.

At this time, add the prawns and cook for about 5 minutes per side, flipping once, until brown and crisp.

Once cooked, remove from the heat and let stand for 2 minutes.

Plate up the trout and prawns and dress with the leftover chimichurri.

Serving this with 1 cup of white rice and 1 cup of veggies adds 9.5g protein; 62.8g carbs; 0.6g fat; 294.6kcal.

CALORIES 488.5KCAL | PROTEIN 62.6G | CARBS 11.6G | FATS 21.3G

Honey & Sesame Seed Salmon with White Rice

This is a tasty Asian infusion that perfectly combines salmon and white rice. The sweetness of the honey and the crunch of the sesame seeds adds a wonderful texture in contrast with the softness of the salmon and rice.

PREP : 10 MINUTES | COOK : 15 MINUTES | SERVES : 3

600g salmon fillets

1 tsp finely diced fresh ginger

2 tbs finely diced shallots

2 tbs honey

2 tsp soy sauce

2 tsp sesame oil

2 tsp olive oil, plus more for cooking

Juice of ½ lime

2 tbs sesame seeds, plus more for garnish

Salt & pepper

Cooked white rice, for serving

Dice your salmon fillets into bite-size pieces or simply cook whole fillets.

Prepare your marinade by mixing together the ginger, shallots, honey, soy sauce, sesame oil, olive oil, lime juice, and sesame seeds.

Coat your frying pan with olive oil and preheat on medium heat.

Fry the salmon for about 5 minutes, until brown. Season with a pinch of salt and pepper.

Drizzle your salmon with half of your marinade and cook for another minute.

Plate your salmon on a bed of rice. Drizzle with the remaining marinade and sprinkle on some extra sesame seeds.

Serving this with 1 cup of white rice and 1 cup of veggies adds 9.5g protein; 62.8g carbs; 0.6g fat; 294.6kcal.

CALORIES 517KCAL | PROTEIN 41.6G | CARBS 14.7G | FATS 32.5G

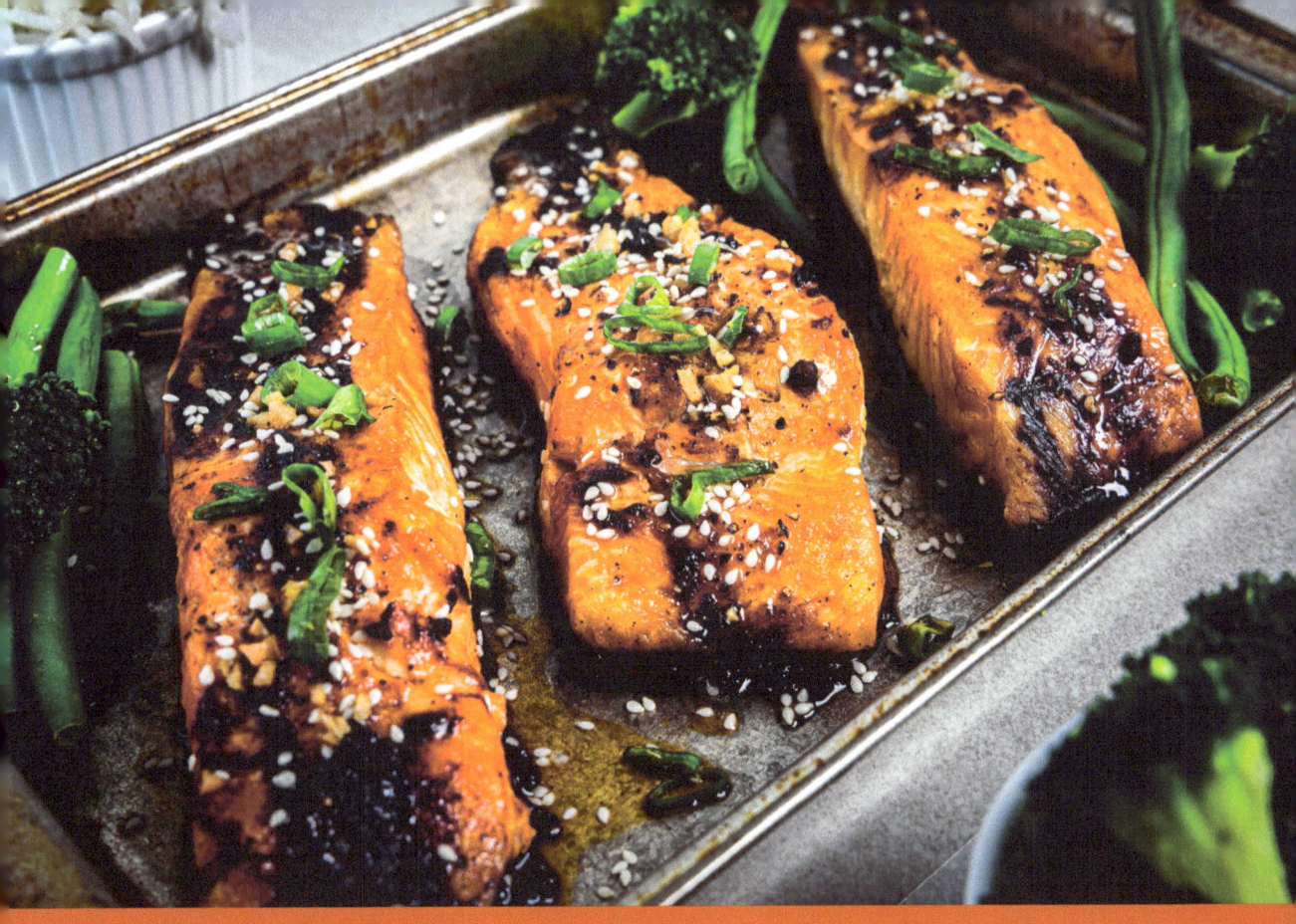

TRY ADDING CHILLI IN THE MARINADE FOR EXTRA FLAVOUR.

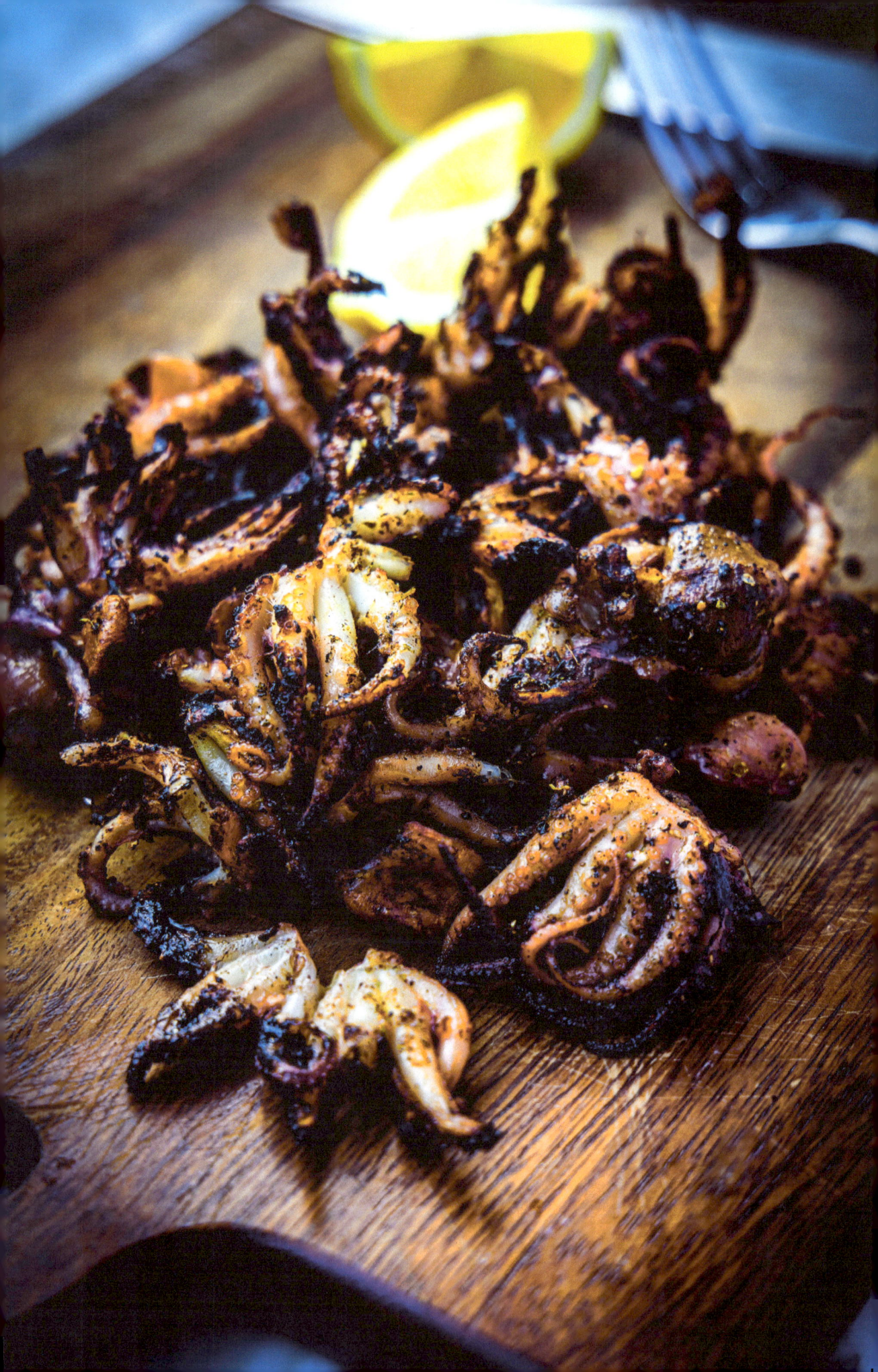

GRILLED BBQ OCTOPUS WITH LEMON & OREGANO

BBQ octopus is famous for that chargrilled flavour. It's best cooked with a Greek-style lemon & oregano marinade. The trick to cooking octopus without it being chewy and rubbery is to tenderize it first before putting it on the BBQ. Then, there's only one way to cook it in my opinion: Greek style!

PREP : OVERNIGHT | COOK : 15 MINUTES | SERVES : 5

1kg octopus

Juice of 2 lemons

3 tbs olive oil

1 tsp salt

1 tsp salt & pepper

1 tbs oregano

Buy baby octopus or full-size and cut into pieces. Make sure the beaks are cut out. My preference is to remove the skin, as it will retain water during tenderising and kill your chances of that charred BBQ finish.

Tenderise the octopus before barbequing by boiling it for 1 to 2 hours. Allow the octopus to cool, then dry it with paper towel and air dry overnight in the fridge. The dryer it is, the more char you will get without overcooking.

Make your marinade by mixing the remaining ingredients in a small mixing bowl. Apply half of this to the octopus in a bowl or plastic bag. Before barbequing, let the octopus rest out of the fridge until it's room temperature.

Cook the octopus on a hot BBQ plate or over charcoals, turning every few minutes. Baste with half of the remaining marinade while it's on the grill, after you've turned the octopus.

Serve while hot, drizzled with the last of the marinade.

BEST SERVED STRAIGHT OFF A HOT BARBEQUE AS A "MEZZE," OR ENTRÉE.

CALORIES 233.1KCAL | PROTEIN 30G | CARBS 5.1G | FATS 10.3G

Chicken & Prawn Long Soup

I love to make this soup on those days when you just want to get warmed up. It's high in protein and a filling meal for a soup.

PREP : 5 MINUTES | COOK : 30 MINUTES | SERVES : 2

1 tbs olive oil for cooking

400g chicken breast, sliced

200g prawns

Pinch of salt & pepper

500ml (2 cups) chicken stock

1 tbs soy sauce

5 cups water

1cm piece of fresh ginger

2 x 60g thin egg noodle nests

1 tsp sesame oil

5 shallots, finely diced

6 snow peas

½ carrot, sliced

Pre heat your pan over medium heat with olive oil.

Add the chicken and prawns to the pan. Season both with salt and pepper. Remove from the pan once golden brown.

Mix together the chicken stock, soy sauce, sesame oil, water, and ginger in a pot and bring to boil. Reduce the heat to low and simmer for 10 minutes to enhance the flavours. Stir the broth occasionally so that nothing sticks to the bottom.

Add your egg noodles to the broth and cook for 3 to 4 minutes.

Once the noodles are cooked, place them in a bowl. Top with the chicken, prawns, and diced shallots. Add broth to your bowl until noodles are covered. Remove the ginger.

Add crunchy vegetables like snow peas and sliced carrot to the soup to serve.

Chicken stock is high in protein with 5.9g per cup and rich in iron. All stock is nutrient-dense and beneficial to our immune system. Its protein content comes from the bones that it's cooked with.

CALORIES 611.2KCAL | PROTEIN 77.8G | CARBS 45.3G | FATS 13.2G

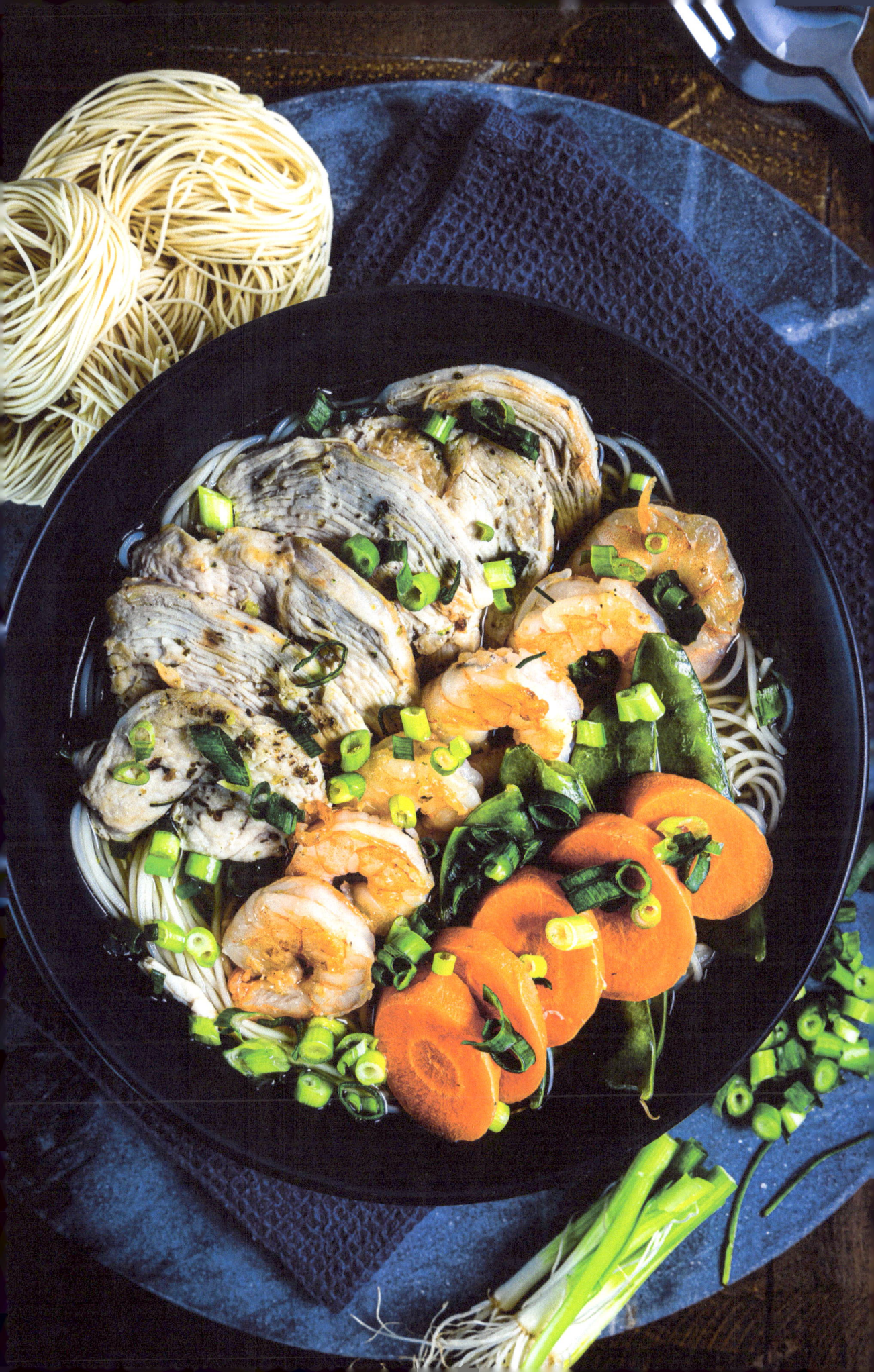

SIDES

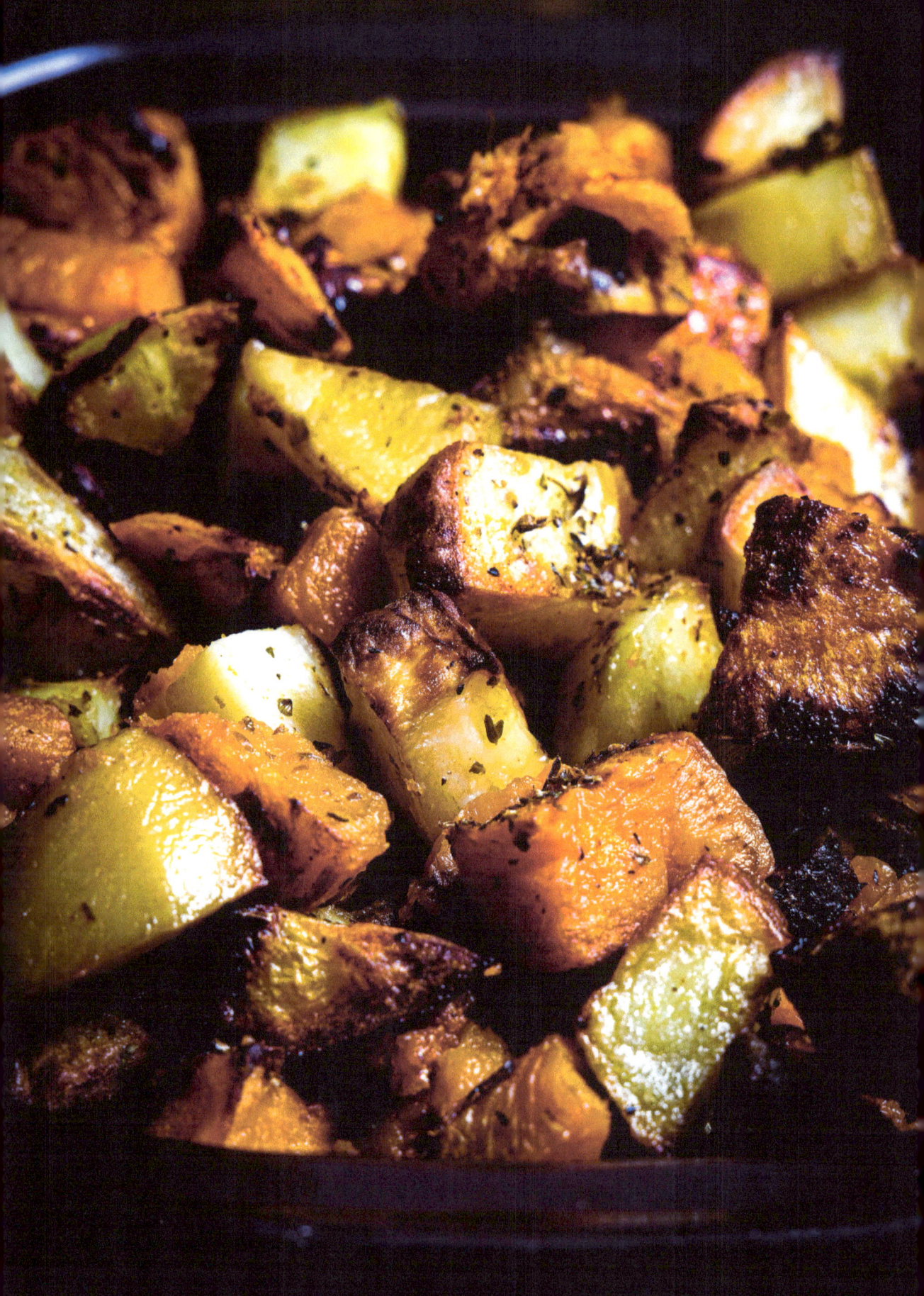

TRY ADDING OTHER HERBS LIKE ROSEMARY AND BASIL.

Baked Potatoes

There's nothing better than crispy and golden potatoes. Potatoes can be baked the fast way where you throw them straight in the oven for 20 minutes or the longer way where you boil and soften them before cooking in the oven to get them crispy. Potatoes can get a bad reputation for being a carbohydrate that contributes to obesity and illness. The truth is, it's the toxic oils they're fried in, the cheese that's added on top, and the butter and cream that's mashed in that causes the health issues. White potatoes and sweet potatoes are nutrient-dense vegetables that satisfy cravings by stabilising blood sugar. They play their role in gut health by promoting good stomach bacteria and starving out destructive bacteria.

PREP : 10 MINUTES | COOK : 60 MINUTES | SERVES : 3 (2 CUPS PER SERVE)

3 large brushed potatoes

1 sweet potato

Juice of ½ lemon

⅓ cup olive oil

1 tbs mixed salt, pepper & oregano

Peel and wash the potatoes to remove all the dirt.

Cut the potatoes into your desired size. Smaller pieces will cook quicker.

Place your potatoes into a pot of boiling water. Simmer for 10 minutes, until the potatoes are soft.

Preheat the oven to 180° to 200°C.

Drain the water and spread the potatoes on a baking tray. The potatoes will have soft and slightly broken edges.

Coat generously with your olive oil and lemon juice. Sprinkle the salt, pepper, and oregano over your potatoes and mix to coat all sides.

Place the tray in the preheated oven. Turn the potatoes occasionally to cook evenly.

Bake for about 45 minutes, until golden.

Serving size = about 2 cups of cooked potatoes
The fastest way to cook potatoes in the oven is to skip the boiling process.

CALORIES 471.4KCAL | PROTEIN 11G | CARBS 62.3G | FATS 19.8G

Boiled Rice

Boiled rice is definitely a weekly staple because it's the quickest carbohydrate to prepare. For the sake of variety, rotate the type of rice you buy. It's healthy and full of energy. Using a rice cooker makes it so easy to cook in bulk, making it easy to cover your meals for the next two days. Leftover rice is perfect for fried rice the next night (see my fried rice recipe on page 81).

PREP : 2 MINUTES | COOK : 10–25 MINUTES | SERVES : 4

2 cups uncooked
(= 4 cups cooked)

White rice

Long & medium grain

Jasmine

Basmati

Brown rice

Couscous

You only need to remember the ratio of rice and water. Check your rice cooker instructions, but the typical ratio is:

1 cup white rice : 1 cup water (or 1 ½ cups water for softer texture)

1 cup brown rice : 1 ½ cups water

Rice Cooker Method: Measure your rice and water into your rice cooker. Set white rice to 10 minutes or brown rice for 20 minutes in your microwave. Alternatively, hit the start button on your electric rice cooker which automatically cooks for roughly the same time.

Stovetop Method: Measure your rice and water into a large pot and bring to a boil. Use the ratios listed in step 1. The reason I don't typically use this method is the extra time is takes to boil and it makes an extra pot to wash. I'm looking for efficiency.

Couscous cooks similarly to rice. Add couscous to boiling water at a 1:1 ratio.

Aim for 1 cup of cooked rice per meal (57g carbohydrates) if you have an average daily activity level.

CALORIES 249.4 KCAL | PROTEIN 4.3G | CARBS 57.6G | FATS 0.2G

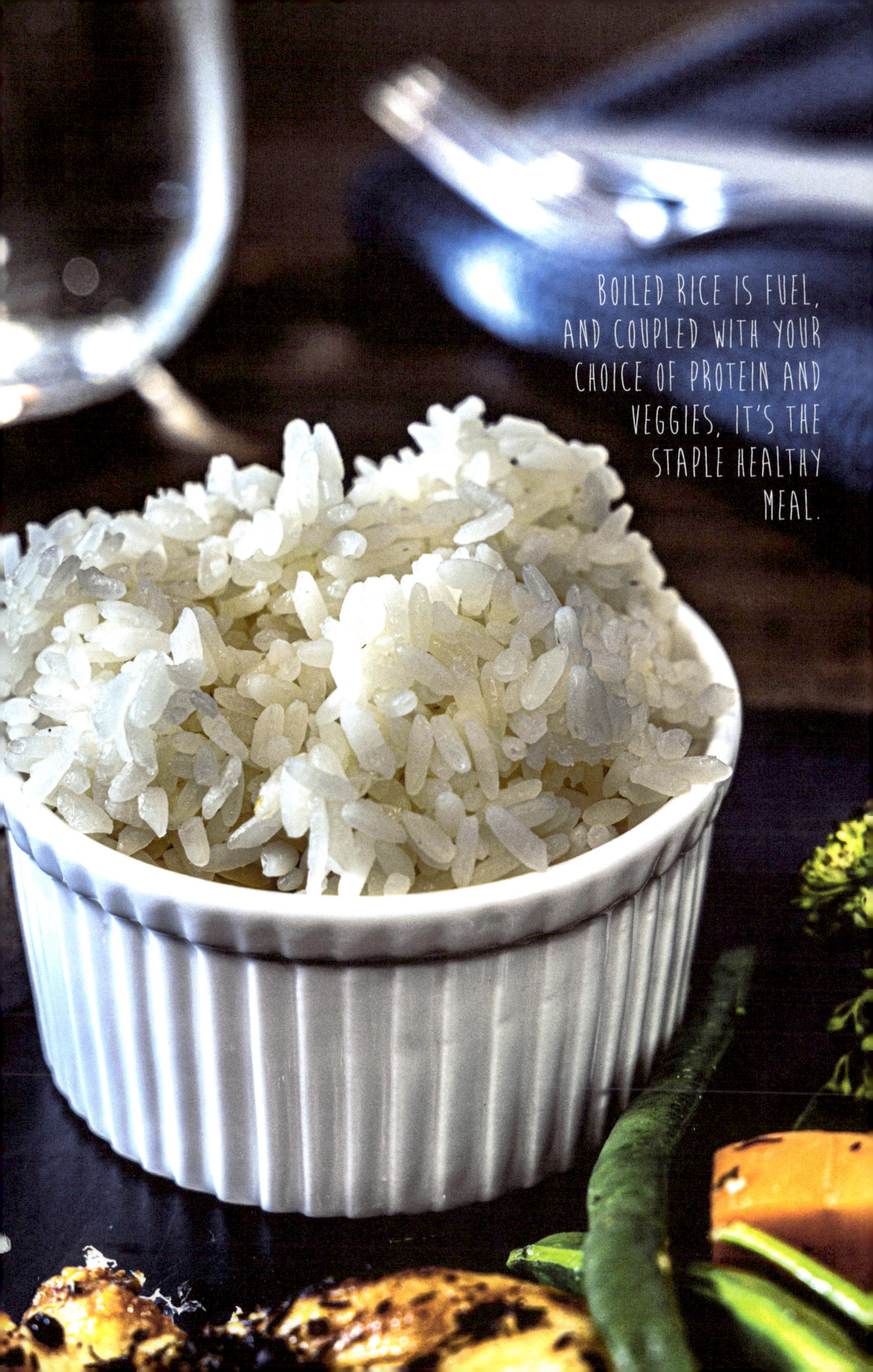

Boiled rice is fuel, and coupled with your choice of protein and veggies, it's the staple healthy meal.

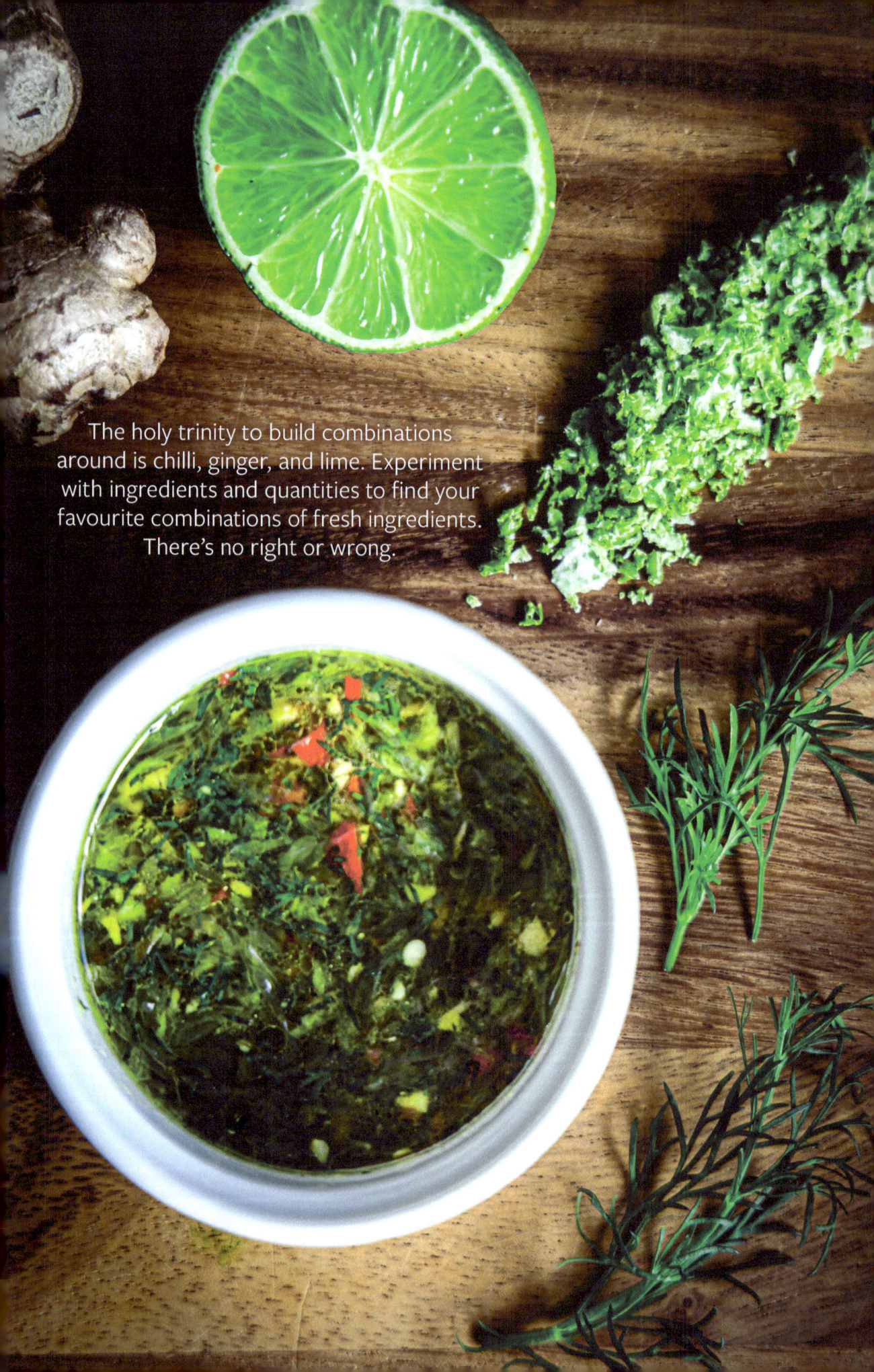

The holy trinity to build combinations around is chilli, ginger, and lime. Experiment with ingredients and quantities to find your favourite combinations of fresh ingredients. There's no right or wrong.

CHIMICHURRI & MARINADES

There are countless varieties of chimichurri and marinades and they deserve a dedicated page. Traditional chimichurri is a sauce or dressing consisting of parsley, garlic, oregano, and olive oil but I choose to make my own version. You will learn over time which flavours go best with fish or pork or chicken. I like that you can jam-pack these with so many fresh herbs that make your taste buds come alive. Experiment with these combinations and come up with your own. You get the flavour and nutrient hit and there's not much pay off with calories.

PREP : 5 MINUTES | COOK : 0 MINUTES | SERVES : 2

Honey & Soy

1 small chilli

1 garlic clove

1 tbs soy sauce

1 tbs honey

1 tsp freshly chopped dill

Garlic & Herbs

1 tbs olive oil

1 tbs mixed freshly chopped mint, basil & parsley

1 small chilli

1 garlic clove

1 tbs honey

Ginger & Herbs

Juice & zest of 1 lime

1 tsp honey

1 tbs olive oil

1 tsp freshly chopped mint

1 tsp freshly chopped dill

1 small chilli

1 tsp minced ginger

Soy & Sesame

1 tbs soy sauce

1 tbs sesame oil

1 small chilli

1 tbs freshly chopped mint & parsley

1 tsp minced ginger

Finely chop your chilli, ginger, garlic and herbs depending on which ingredients you're using.

Grate your lime zest.

Add a pinch of salt.

Mix the ingredients in a bowl or use a mortar & pestle to crush and mix.

Dress your food before and after cooking.

CALORIES 109.3KCAL | PROTEIN 0.2G | CARBS 11.6G | FATS 6.9G

GUACAMOLE

Do you love avocados but they ripen faster than you eat them? Never again fear an oversupply of avocados—guacamole will solve this problem for you. It has such a fresh and explosive flavour with the lime and chilli that you can't help but go for more and more!

PREP : 10 MINUTES | COOK : 0 MINUTES | SERVES : 6

3 avocados

1 chilli, finely chopped

1 tsp finely chopped fresh ginger

⅓ cup freshly chopped parsley, plus more for garnish

Juice of 2 limes

1 tbs olive oil

¾ punnet baby tomatoes, diced

Remove the avocado from its skin and mash in a mixing bowl with a fork.

Add the chilli, ginger, and parsley.

Squeeze the juice of both limes into the bowl. Mix in the olive oil as well.

Chop the baby tomatoes into quarters. Mix half of the tomatoes with the avocado. The remainder can be placed on top to dress the guacamole before serving. Sprinkle a little more parsley on top to serve.

Each serving is 3 tbs.

Use avocados that are soft and ripe. If they are overly ripe then the guacamole will taste off. If they are too hard then you won't be able to mash them. Keep your eye on your avocados to make this at the right time.

CALORIES 188G | PROTEIN 2.1G | CARBS 1.7G | FATS 19.2G

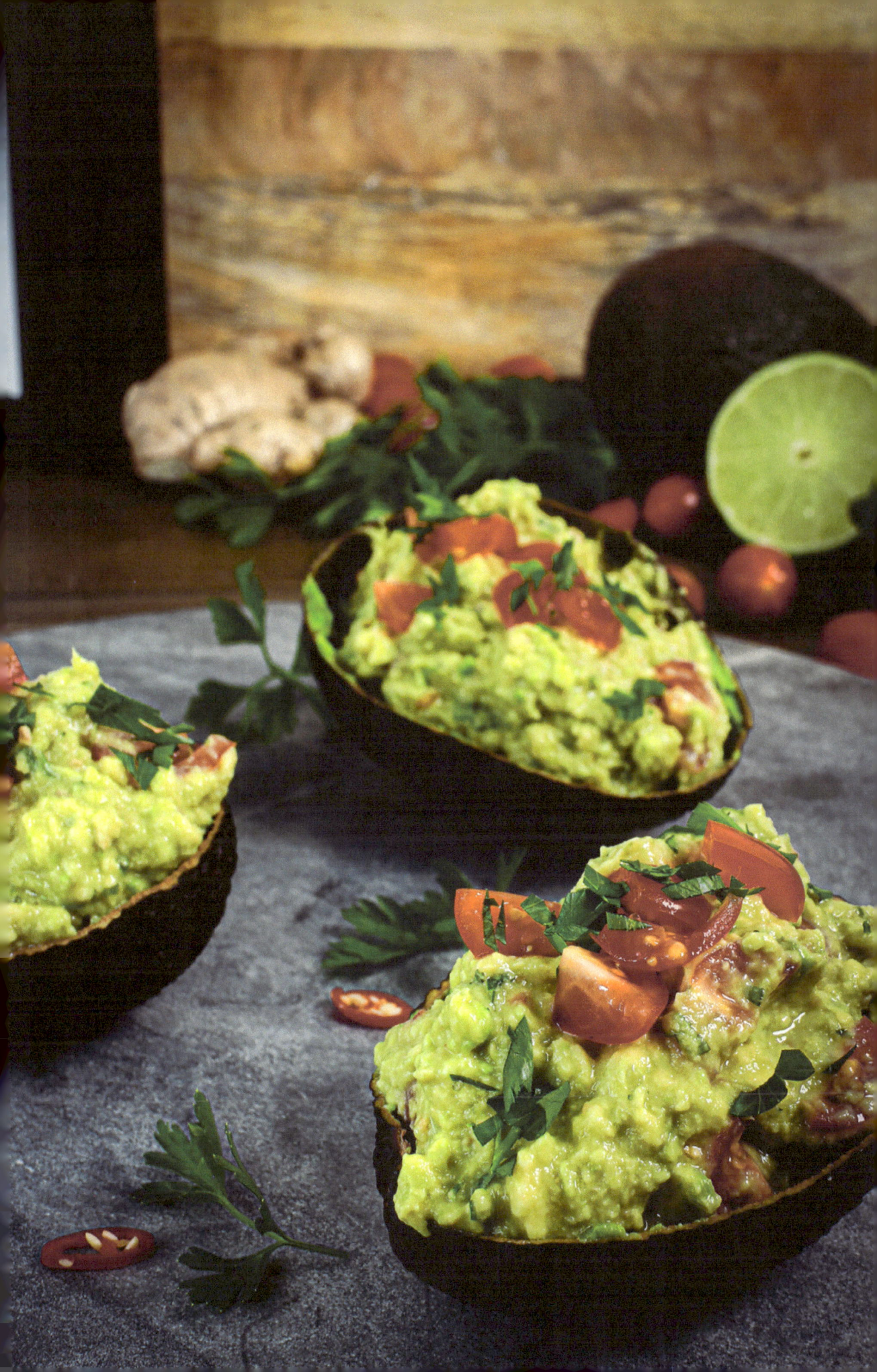

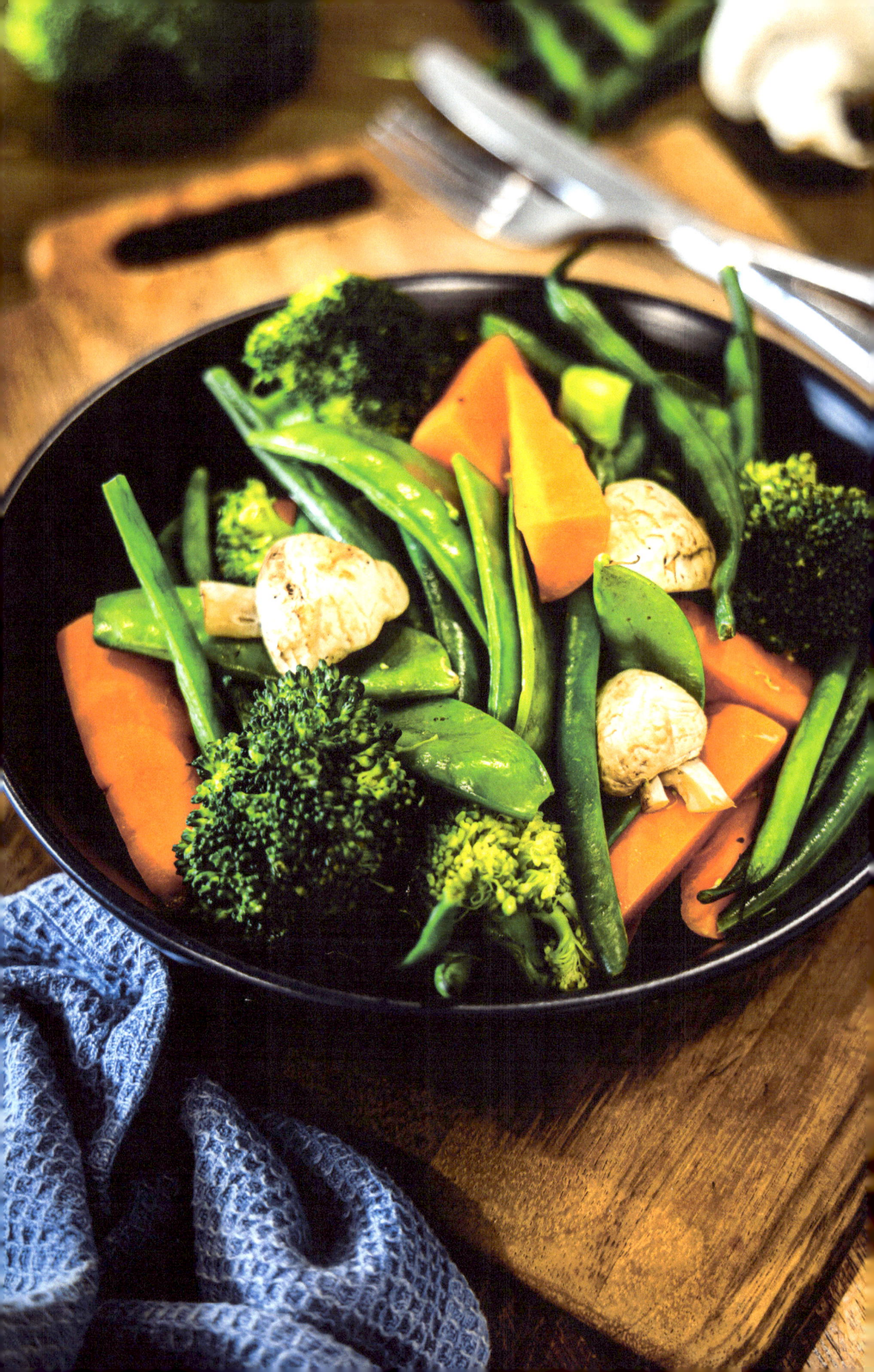

STEAMED VEGETABLES

Steamed vegetables are a fast side dish which should help get them onto your plate more frequently. The best method to avoid ending up with soggy veggies is to use a steamer basket over boiling water. The cooking time will vary slightly between vegetables. The more dense they are, the more cooking time required. Broccoli and carrots will take a couple more minutes than thinner veggies like green beans.

PREP : 10 MINUTES | COOK : 8 MINUTES | SERVES : 3

- 2 cups broccoli florets
- 1 carrot
- 1 cup green beans
- Mushrooms & snow peas (optional)

Bring a cup of water to boil in a pot on medium heat and place the steamer basket on top.

While your water is coming to a boil, cut your vegetables into even, bite-size pieces.

Add your vegetables to the steamer basket and cover with a lid. Add them in order of required cooking time so they complete cooking at the same time. For example, broccoli and carrots should go in first for 2 minutes before adding the greens so they all finish cooking in about 6 to 8 minutes.

Test the veggies for readiness by poking with a knife or tasting a piece.

To remove from the heat, tilt the lid away from you to avoid the steam and use a tea towel to grab the handles of the steamer basket.

VEGETABLES ARE A FIBROUS CARBOHYDRATE WHICH MEANS THEY WILL MAKE YOU FEEL FULL. EATING THEM FIRST FROM YOUR PLATE SHOULD HELP OVER EATING OTHER THINGS.

CALORIES 45.2G | PROTEIN 5.2G | CARBS 5.2G | FATS 0.4G

TOMATO PASTA SAUCE

This is your go-to tomato pasta sauce when you need something quick for dinner. It's perfect for adding flavour to a piece of chicken breast or mixing through pasta. The base of the sauce (canned crushed tomatoes, olive oil, and garlic) is there for you to mix and match your favourite herbs.

PREP : 5 MINUTES | COOK : 25 MINUTES | SERVES : 3

3 tbs olive oil for cooking

3 garlic cloves, finely diced

3 mushrooms, diced

1 small chilli, finely diced

410g can crushed tomatoes

1 tbs freshly chopped parsley

1 tbs freshly chopped basil

1 cup pitted olives

Heat the olive oil in your pan on medium heat.

Add the garlic, chilli, and mushrooms and add to the pan for a minute to brown.

Add the can of tomatoes and the remainder of the olive oil.

Reduce the heat to medium-low and simmer for another 20 minutes, until thickened.

Mix in the herbs and olives and add a pinch of salt and pepper. Cook for 1 minute.

Serve with pasta or add to your protein. The best option is to add your cooked pasta straight to the sauce. Drain the cooked pasta without rinsing with clean water. Add 3 servings of pasta straight to the pasta sauce in the pan still on low heat. Mix well for 2 minutes. The starch remaining on the pasta helps the sauce stick.

CALORIES 147 KCAL | PROTEIN 1.5G | CARBS 4.5G | FATS 13.7G

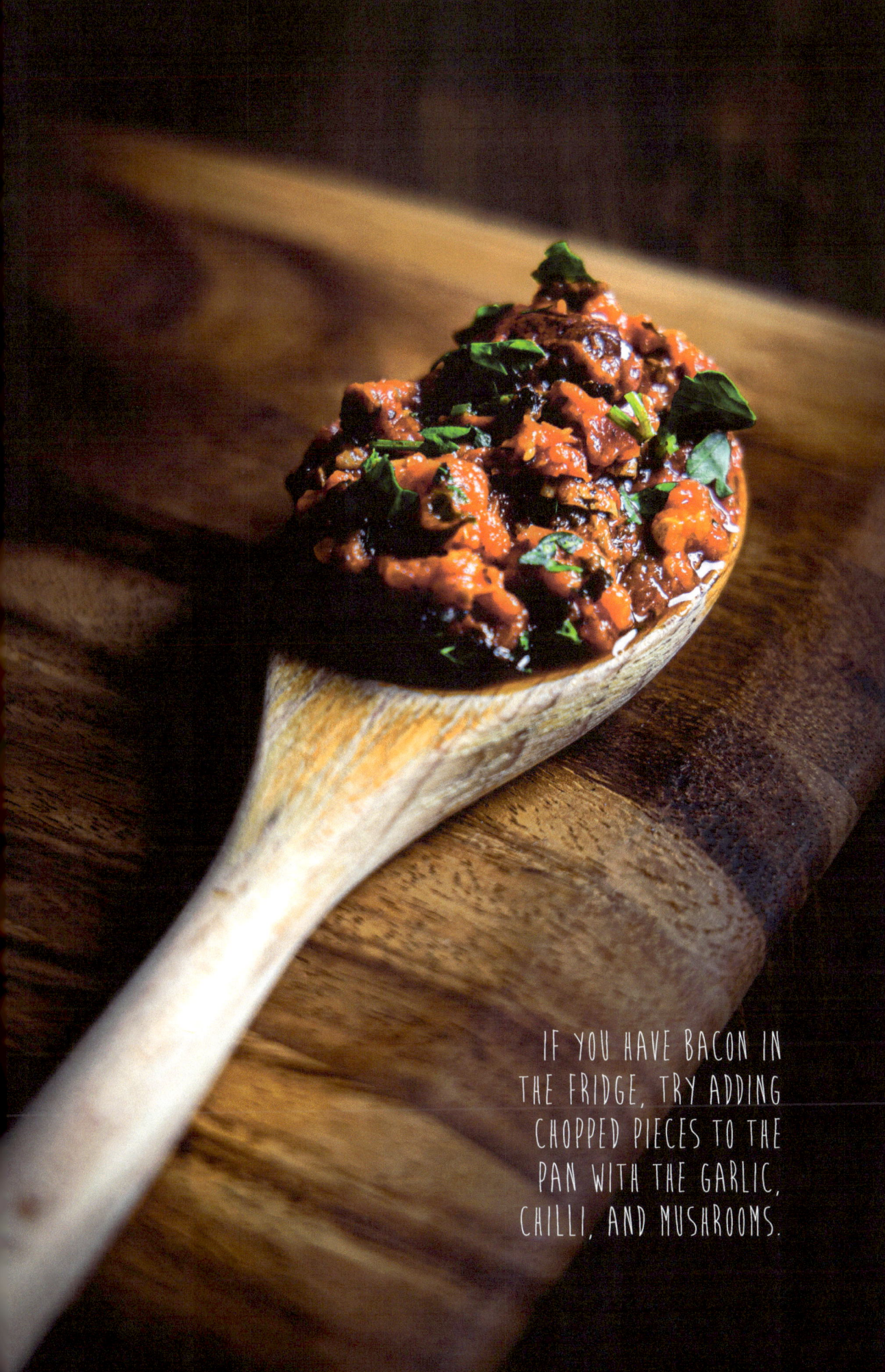

If you have bacon in the fridge, try adding chopped pieces to the pan with the garlic, chilli, and mushrooms.

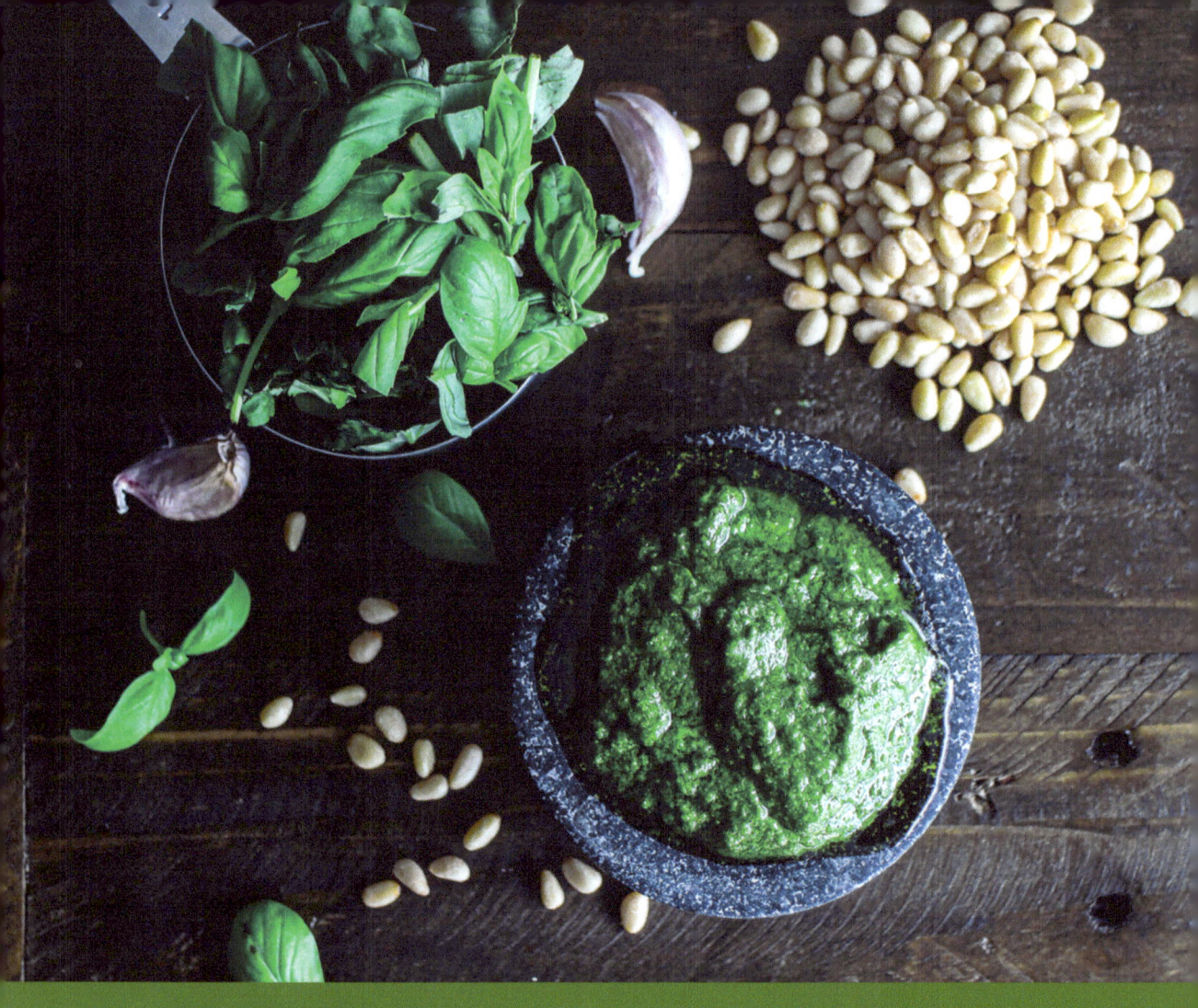

Try this with ¾ cup of parmesan cheese mixed in.

Pesto Pasta Sauce

I alternate between tomato pasta sauce and pesto. When you know how to make pesto as well, you should not need to ever go back to bottle pasta sauces. Here you get the freshest and healthiest ingredients that pack more flavour than off the shelf. It also has less sugar and fat as well.

PREP : 5 MINUTES | COOK : 0 MINUTES | SERVES : 8

½ cup roasted pine nuts

2 cups basil

2 cloves of garlic

½ cup olive oil

Juice of ½ lemon

Pinch of salt & pepper

Add the pine nuts, basil, and garlic to your bullet blender (a food processor is better if you have one). Blend until finely chopped.

Add the olive oil, lemon juice, salt, and pepper and blend to a paste.

This quantity is enough to mix through a cooked bag (500g) of pasta. One bag has 8 cups of pasta. Alternatively, store in the fridge for up to 5 days in an air-tight sealed jar.

CALORIES 179.2KCAL | PROTEIN 1.1G | CARBS 0.5G | FATS 19.2G

Greek Salad

A Greek salad has several variations, but I say the classic ingredients include tomatoes, cucumber, capsicum, olives, and fetta cheese. Splash some lemon juice and olive oil on top and your dressing is done!

PREP : 5 MINUTES | COOK : 0 MINUTES | SERVES : 2

2 tomatoes

1 cucumber

⅓ capsicum

Juice of ½ lemon

2 tbs olive oil

½ tsp freshly chopped basil

½ tsp freshly chopped parsley

10–20 olives

1 block of fetta cheese

Cut the tomatoes and cucumber into bite-size pieces.

Cut the capsicum into long, thin strips.

Mix everything in a bowl with your lemon juice, olive oil, and olives.

Add bite-size pieces of fetta on top.

Add thin strips of onion if desired.

CALORIES 212.2 KCAL | PROTEIN 0.8G | CARBS 2.3G | FATS 22.2G

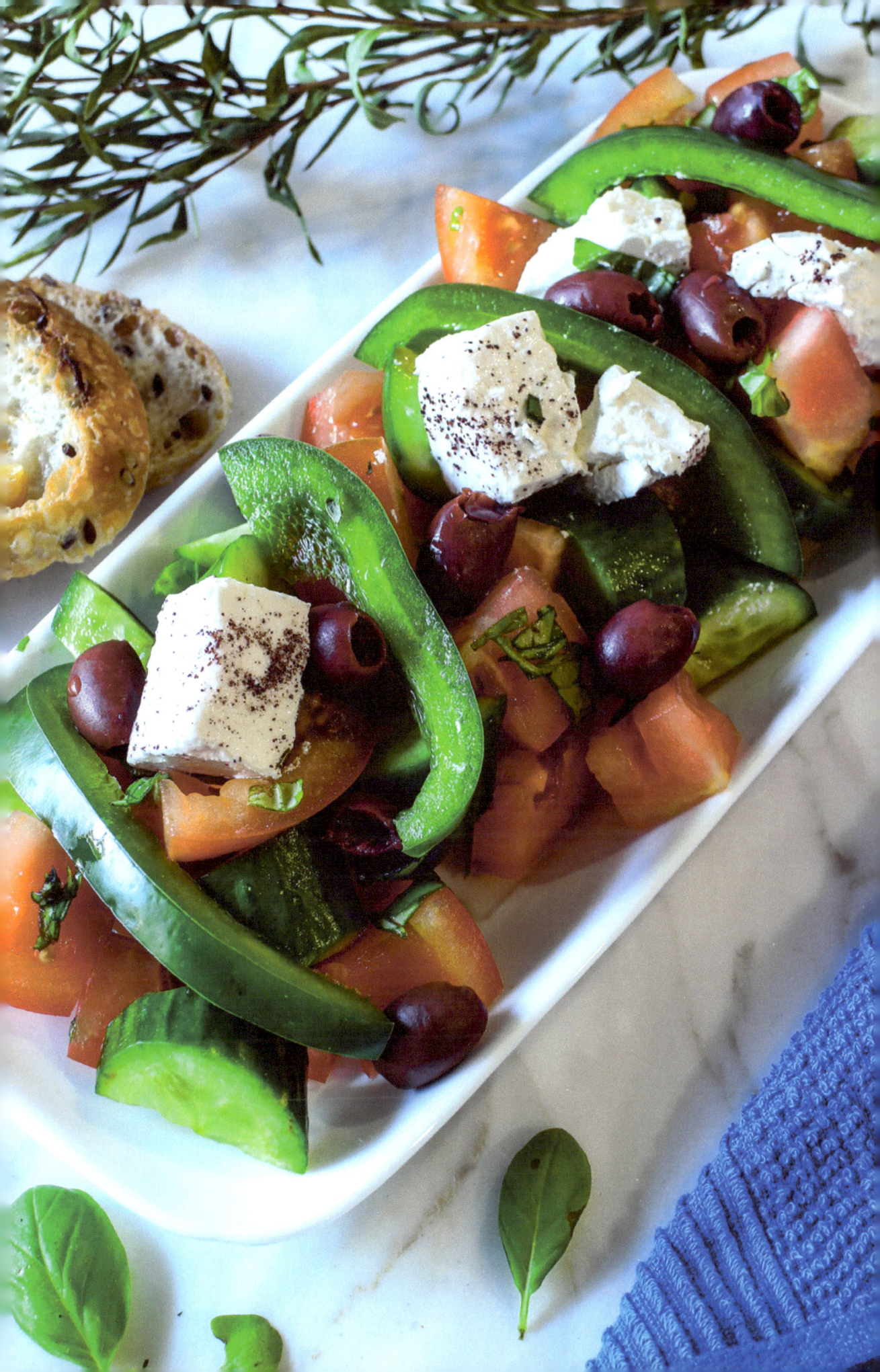

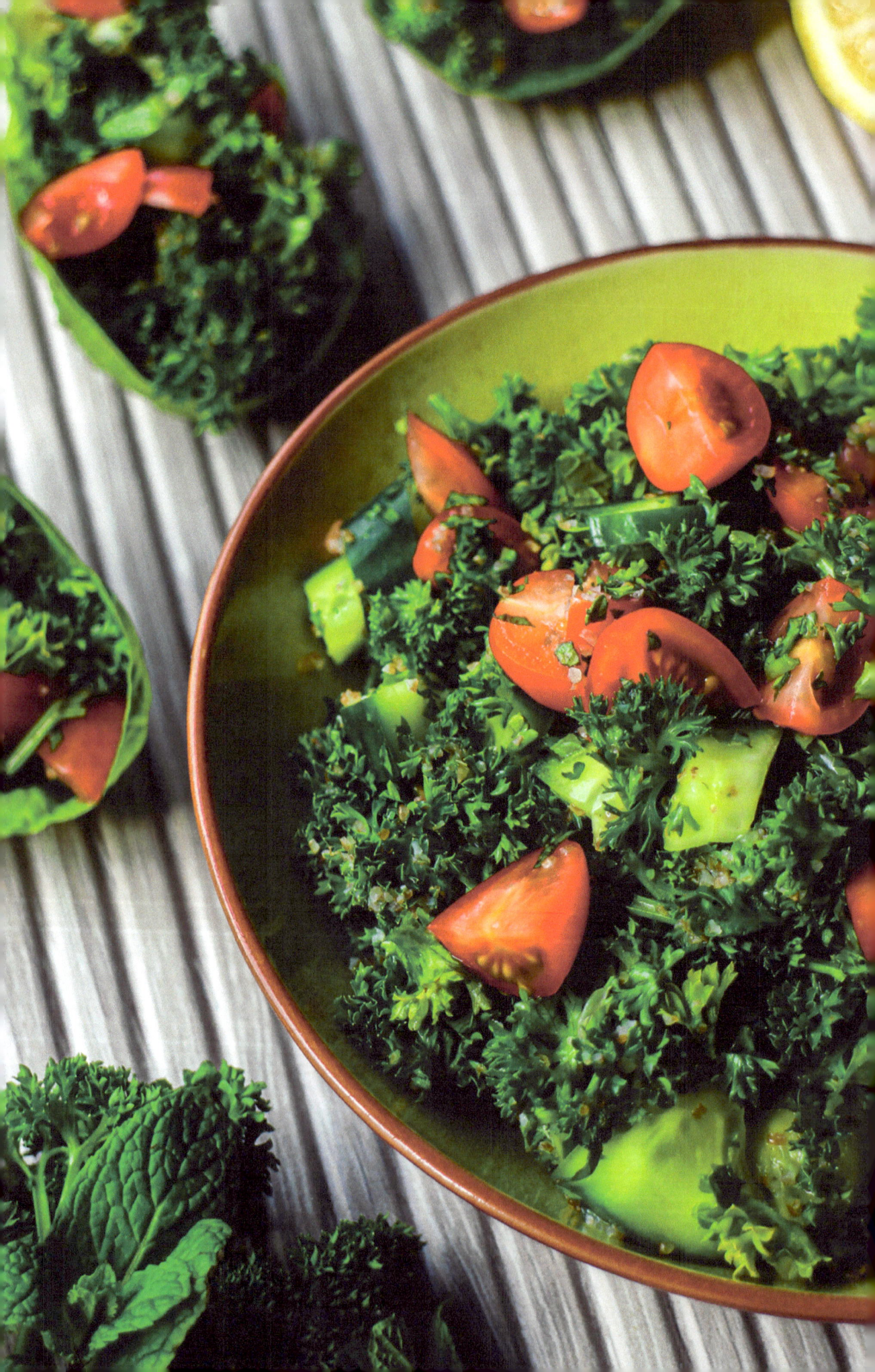

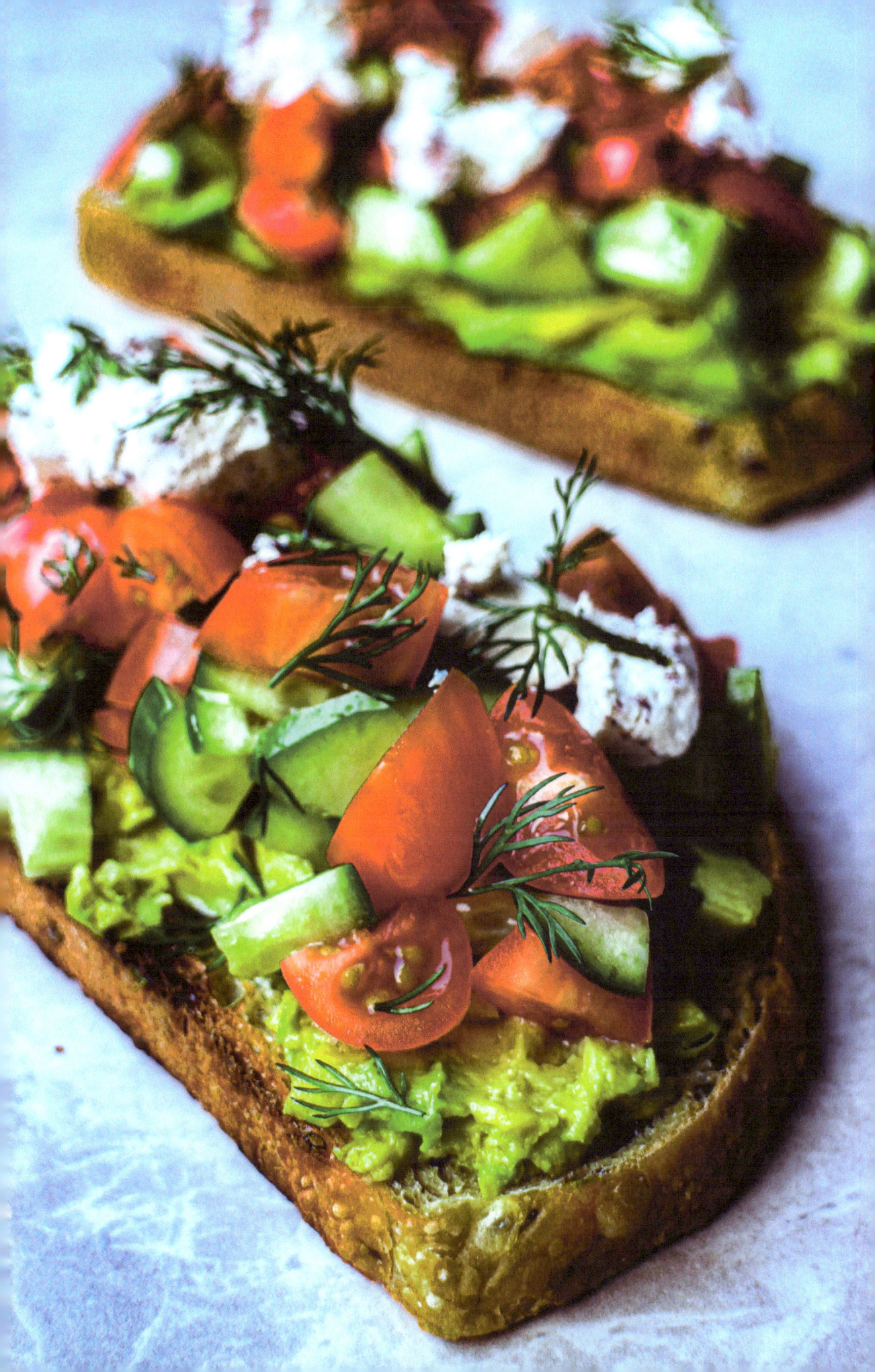

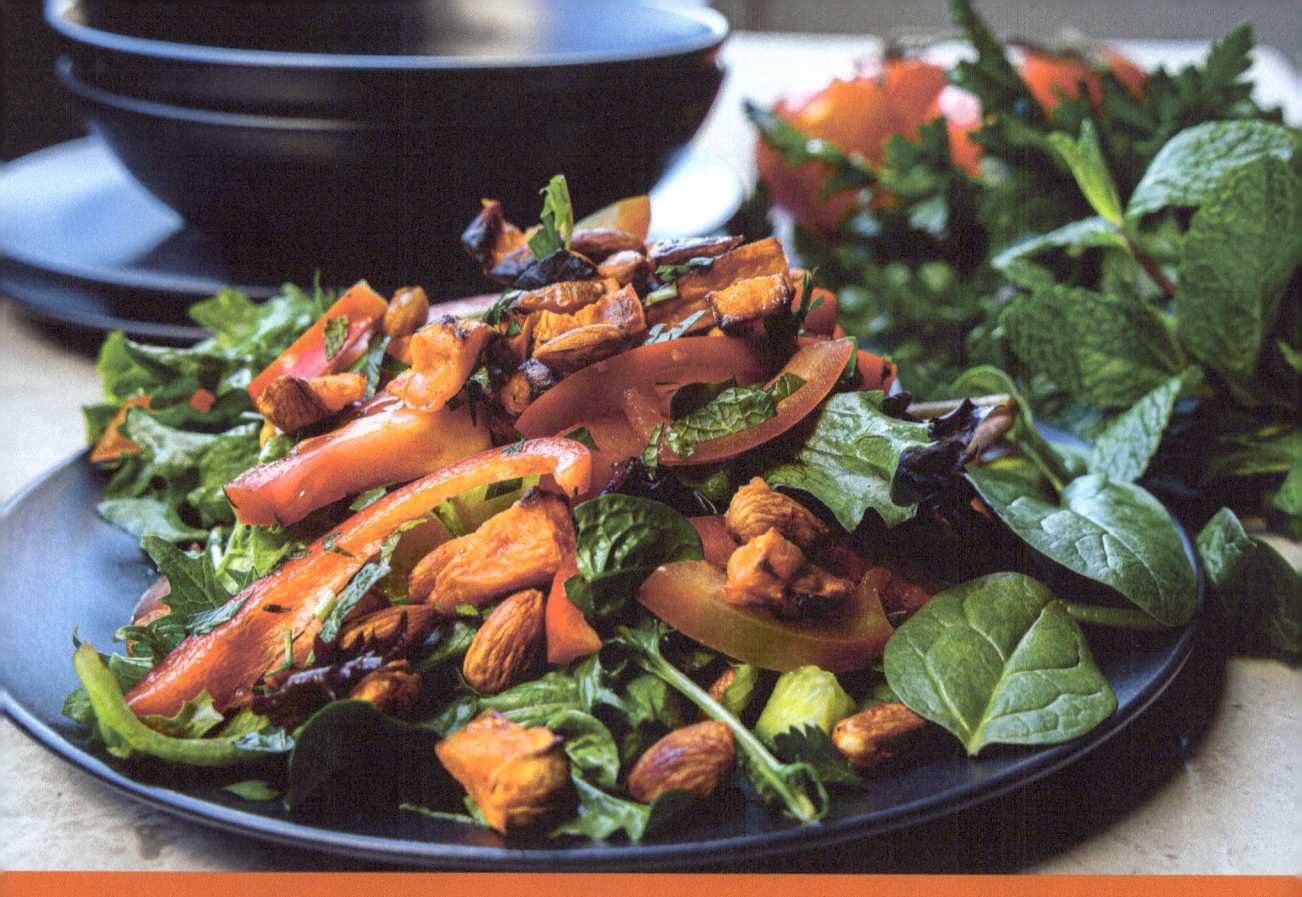

Did you know spinach is one of the most calorically light but nutrient dense foods and has 5.5g protein per cup?

Green Leafy Salad

Salads do not need to be overly complicated. The calories in a salad are next to zero and you can almost consider them free calories. Salads are good for you for their antioxidant properties, and being fibrous carbohydrates means you can fill up on them without paying the price of overeating calories. Lemon and olive oil salad dressing is a simple and healthy option. This salad variation with the almonds and sweet potato will pack a little more energy if you want to reduce other carbohydrates in your meal.

PREP : 10 MINUTES | COOK : 30 MINUTES | SERVES : 4

1 cup chopped sweet potato

½ cup almonds

1 tomato

1 cucumber

½ capsicum

4 cups leafy greens

1 tbs freshly chopped parsley

1 tbs freshly chopped mint

1 tbs olive oil

Juice of ½ lemon

Preheat your oven to 180°C. Bake the sweet potatoes for about 30 minutes, until tender.

Toast the almonds in a pan on medium heat to bring out their nutty flavour. Flip the almonds every few minutes. Remove from heat after 10 minutes.

Cut your tomato, cucumber, and capsicum as you like and throw in a large bowl with the leafy greens, parsley, and mint.

Let the potato cool for couple of minutes and add to your salad with the olive oil and lemon juice.

Mix thoroughly and serve.

CALORIES 228.1KCAL | PROTEIN 7.1G | CARBS 20G | FATS 13.3G

SNACKS

YOGURT, BERRIES & MUESLI

This is the perfect alternative to ice cream for a late-night snack. I mix the yogurt with protein powder for flavour and extra protein. The sweetness of the berries and muesli gives me that sugar fix that I sometimes crave. I don't worry about the sugar at night because it fuels me for my early-morning workouts. The antioxidant benefits from the fruit are something I don't want to miss out on either.

PREP : 5 MINUTES | COOK : 0 MINUTES | SERVES : 1

4 tbs low-sugar Greek yogurt

1 scoop whey protein powder

½ cup mixed raspberries, blueberries, and/or strawberries

½ cup muesli

1 passionfruit

Add the yogurt and protein powder into a bowl. Stir thoroughly. Chocolate whey goes well with vanilla or plain yogurt.

Add your berries then add the muesli on top. I use cocoa-flavoured muesli.

Scatter your passionfruit over the muesli.

SOMETIMES I USE COCOA POWDER AS A SUBSTITUTE TO PROTEIN POWDER FOR VARIETY.

CALORIES 470KCAL | PROTEIN 39.5G | CARBS 43G | FATS 15.5G

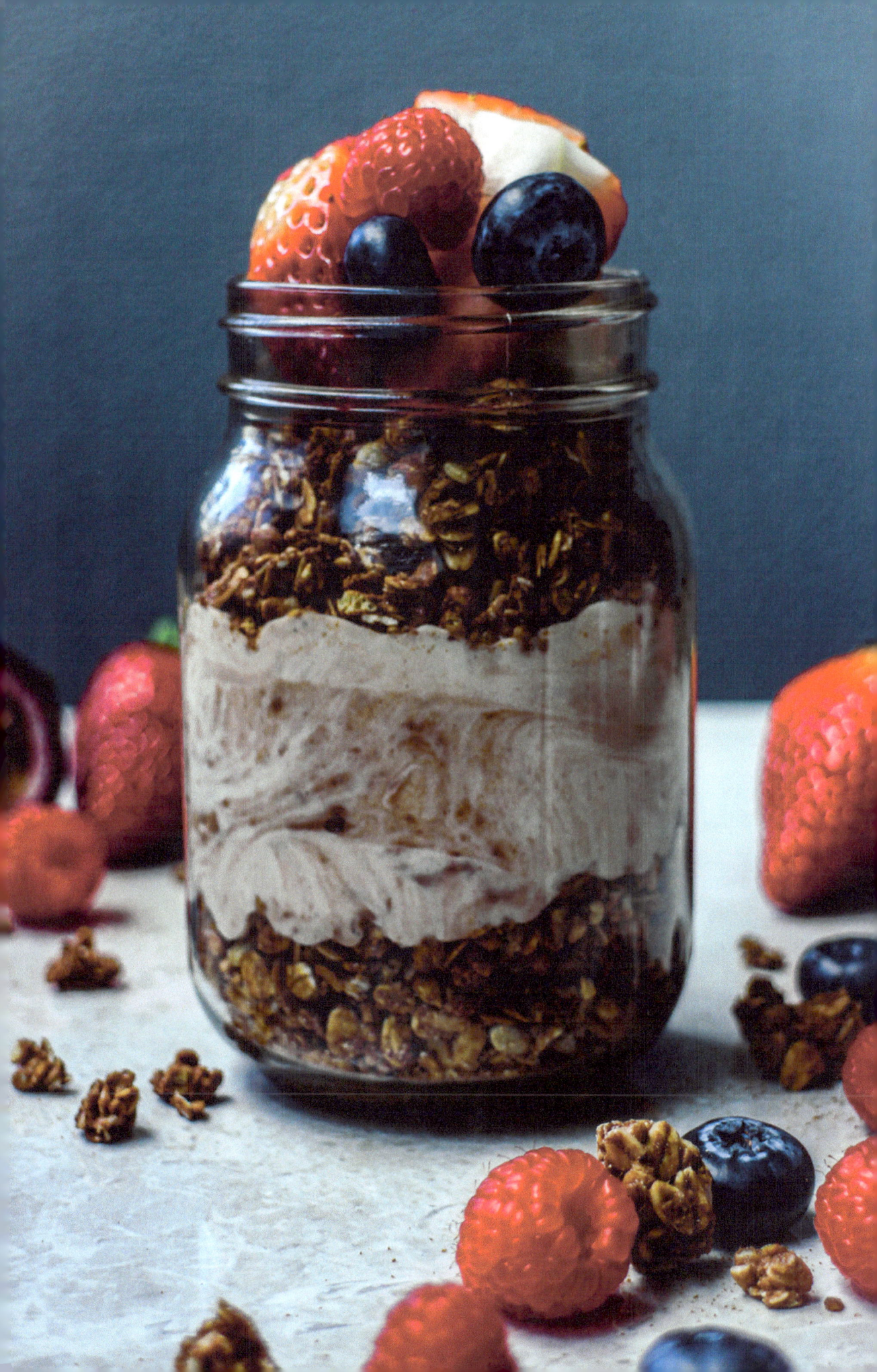

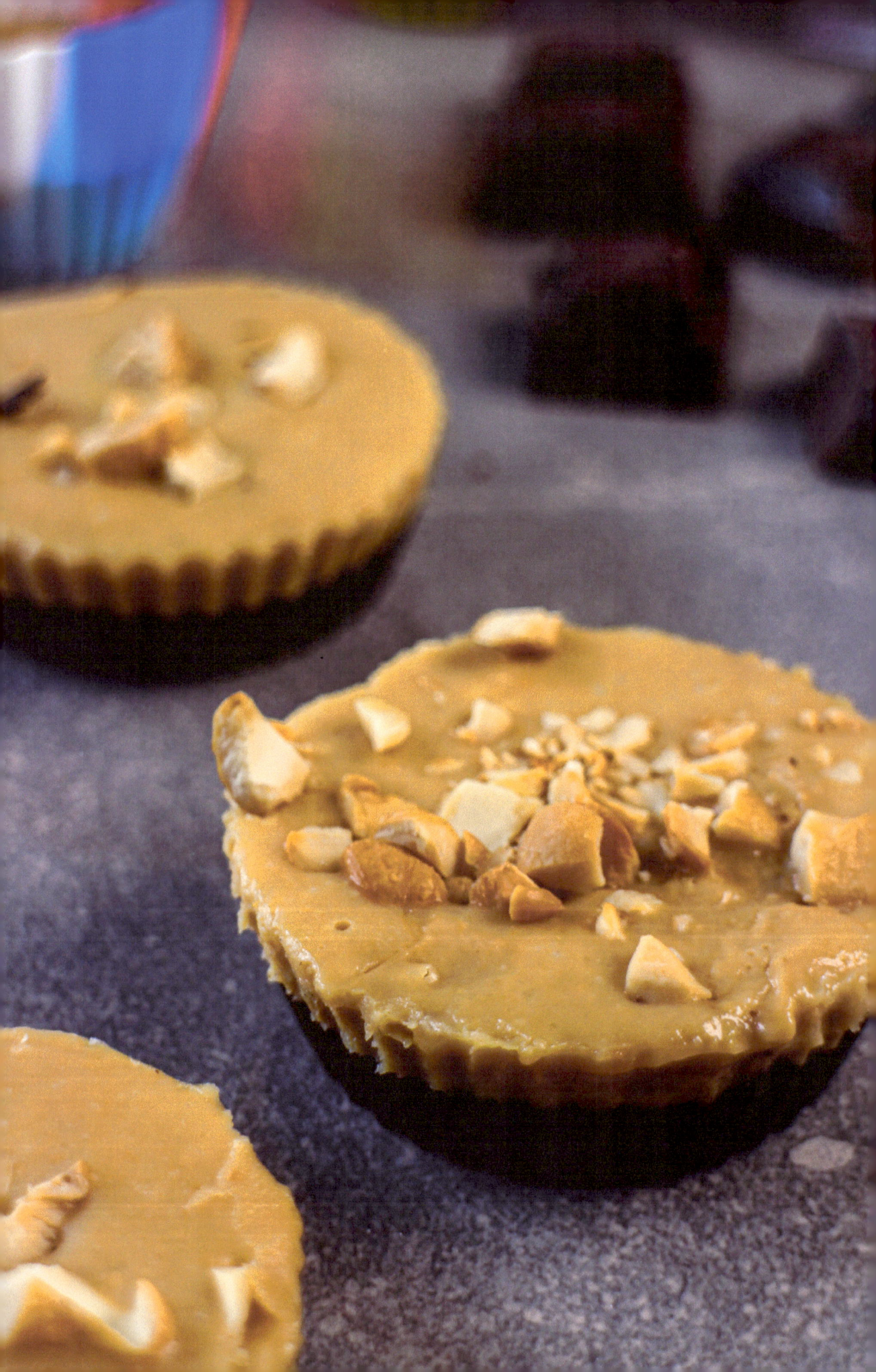

DARK CHOCOLATE & PEANUT BUTTER CUPS

This is a high-energy snack that you shouldn't feel guilty having. It's loaded with healthy fats and energy for your busy day. Dark chocolate boasts antioxidant properties and several health benefits.

PREP : 2-3 HOURS | COOK : 0 MINUTES | SERVES : 2 CUPS

180g block dark chocolate (70% cocoa)

1 tsp honey

2 tbs peanut butter

2 tbs coconut oil

Pinch of salt

1 tbs crushed cashews

Melt the chocolate in the microwave in 30-second intervals, stirring in between so it doesn't burn, for a total of 2 minutes, or until fully melted.

Stir in the honey.

Pour 1 tbs of chocolate into individual baking cups and spread evenly to all sides. I use reusable silicon baking cups that peel away easily later.

Freeze for 10 minutes until the chocolate is just hard.

Meanwhile, mix the peanut butter, coconut oil, and salt in a small bowl until creamy.

Remove the chocolate from the freezer and add a layer of the peanut butter/coconut oil mixture.

Sprinkle a pinch of crushed cashews on top of each cup.

Set this in the freezer for a few hours or overnight and keep in the fridge after that.

SHOUT OUT TO ROSS EDGLEY AND THE WORLD'S FITTEST BOOK FOR THIS RECIPE.

CALORIES 120KCAL | PROTEIN 2.7G | CARBS 5.0G | FATS 10.0G

SMOOTHIES & JUICES

Banana & Protein Smoothie

This shake is my go-to meal replacement. It's full of energy in the form of carbs and healthy fats as well as high in protein with a scoop of whey and an egg. It's the most convenient way to get quick calories in when you're running out the door. Smoothies are the best way to bump up your intake of superfoods like greens, psyllium husk, and flaxseed. Using frozen bananas is the secret to making this smoothie cold and creamy. Using ice can give it a fluffy texture as well.

PREP : 5 MINUTES | COOK : 0 MINUTES | SERVES : 1

1 ½ frozen bananas

1 scoop chocolate whey protein

1 egg

¼ cup rolled oats

½–1 tsp greens superfood powder

1 tbs peanut butter

1 tbs honey

½ tsp cinnamon

1 tbs cocoa powder

1 tbs psyllium husk

Water

Add all the ingredients to your bullet blender. Throw in the whole egg, including the shell after washing it thoroughly. It's an unusual trick I learned from the great Arnold Schwarzenegger. (Egg shells are rich in calcium and one shell provides twice the daily recommended dose.)

Fill your blender to the limit with cold water. Blend.

Psyllium husk and flaxseed powder are interchangeable, as both are high in fibre and loaded with nutrients. Psyllium husk is a natural laxative. Flaxseed contains healthy omega 3 fatty acid which helps with good heart health. Remember, foods high in fibre slow digestion and makes you feel fuller for longer so you have less chance of overeating.

Dates are a perfect addition to this smoothie for added sweetness. Just watch the added carbs from the dates.

CALORIES 701.9 KCAL | PROTEIN 49.4G | CARBS 79.5G | FATS 20.7G

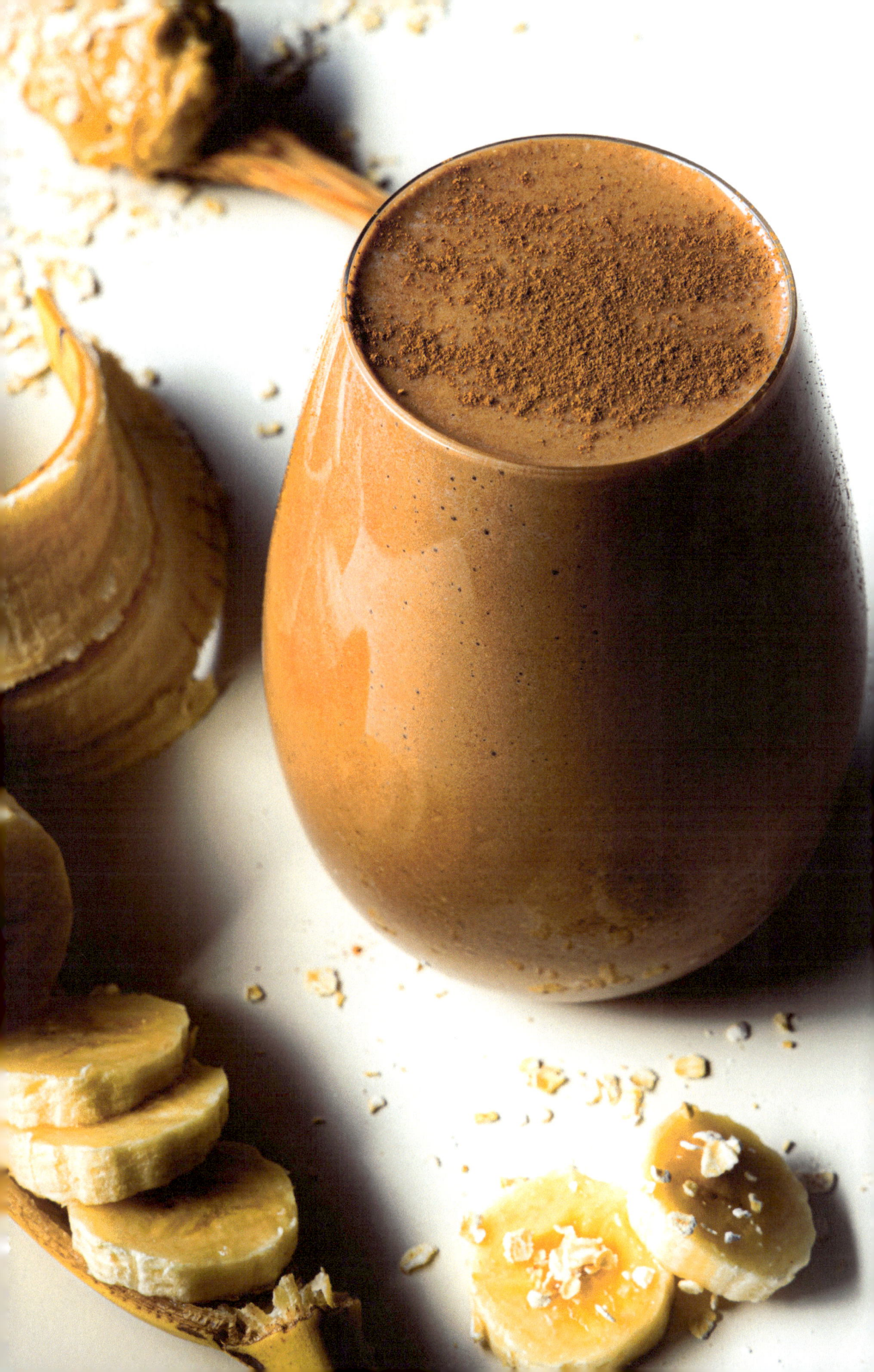

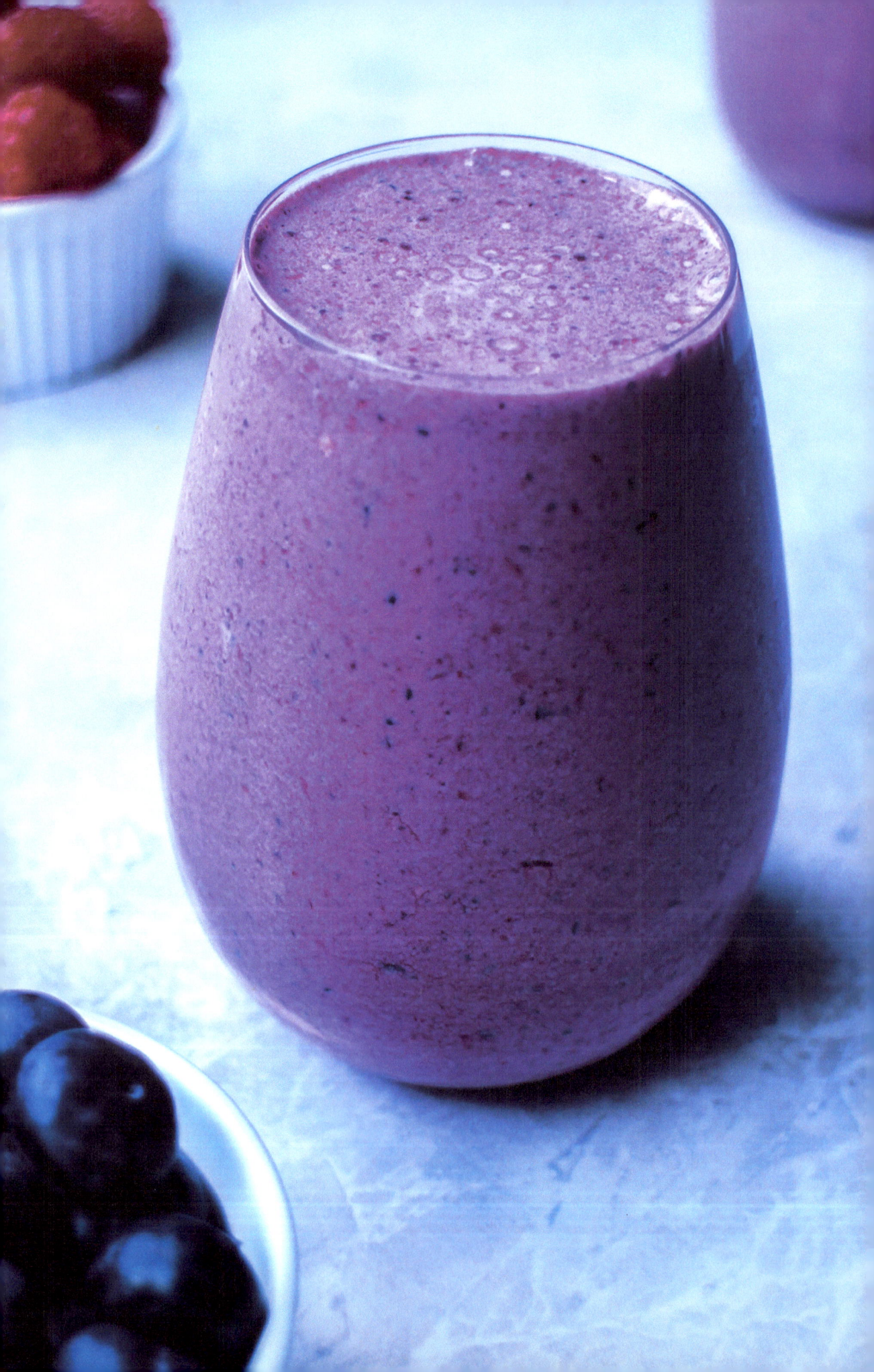

Mixed Berries Smoothie

When you want something cold and refreshing, try this smoothie. This drink is high in antioxidants and fibre and adds a wide variety of superfoods to your diet. With lots of protein, this is a great post-workout drink, and the simple sugars in the berries are fast-acting to replenish the energy stores from your exercise.

PREP : 5 MINUTES | COOK : 0 MINUTES | SERVES : 1

1 cup frozen mixed berries

1 scoop chocolate whey protein

1 egg

¼ cup rolled oats

½–1 tsp greens superfood powder

1–2 tbs coconut butter

1 tsp honey

½ tsp cinnamon

1 tsp cocoa powder

1 tbs psyllium husk

Water

Add all the ingredients to your bullet blender. Throw in the whole egg including the shell (thoroughly washed) for a dose of calcium.

Fill your blender to the limit with cold water. Blend.

There are no set rules with this smoothie. Just throw in any superfoods powder you desire. Limit the quantity of green superfood powder, though, as it can be overpowering.

CALORIES 484.5KCAL | PROTEIN 35.4G | CARBS 53.1G | FATS 14.5G

DATES & GREENS SUPERFOOD SMOOTHIE

Dates are a natural sweetener and make a delicious protein smoothie to satisfy your sweet tooth. They are full of fibre and this smoothie leaves you feeling full for hours. It's a little lighter than the banana shake on page 124, but still sweet and satisfying.

PREP : 5 MINUTES | COOK : 0 MINUTES | SERVES : 1

5 dates

1 frozen banana

1 scoop vanilla whey protein

1 egg

¼ cup rolled oats

1 tsp greens superfood powder

1 tsp honey

½ tsp cinnamon

1 tsp psyllium husk

Water

Add all the ingredients to your bullet blender and blend well. The dates will take a few extra seconds.

Substitute water with coconut water as a natural source of vitamins, minerals, and electrolytes.

Adding half a frozen avocado adds an even smoother and creamier texture to your smoothie.

SUBSTITUTE PSYLLIUM HUSK FOR FLAXSEED POWDER OR SIMPLY USE IT IN ADDITION TO THE FLAXSEED.

CALORIES 552 KCAL | PROTEIN 42.4G | CARBS 74G | FATS 9.6G

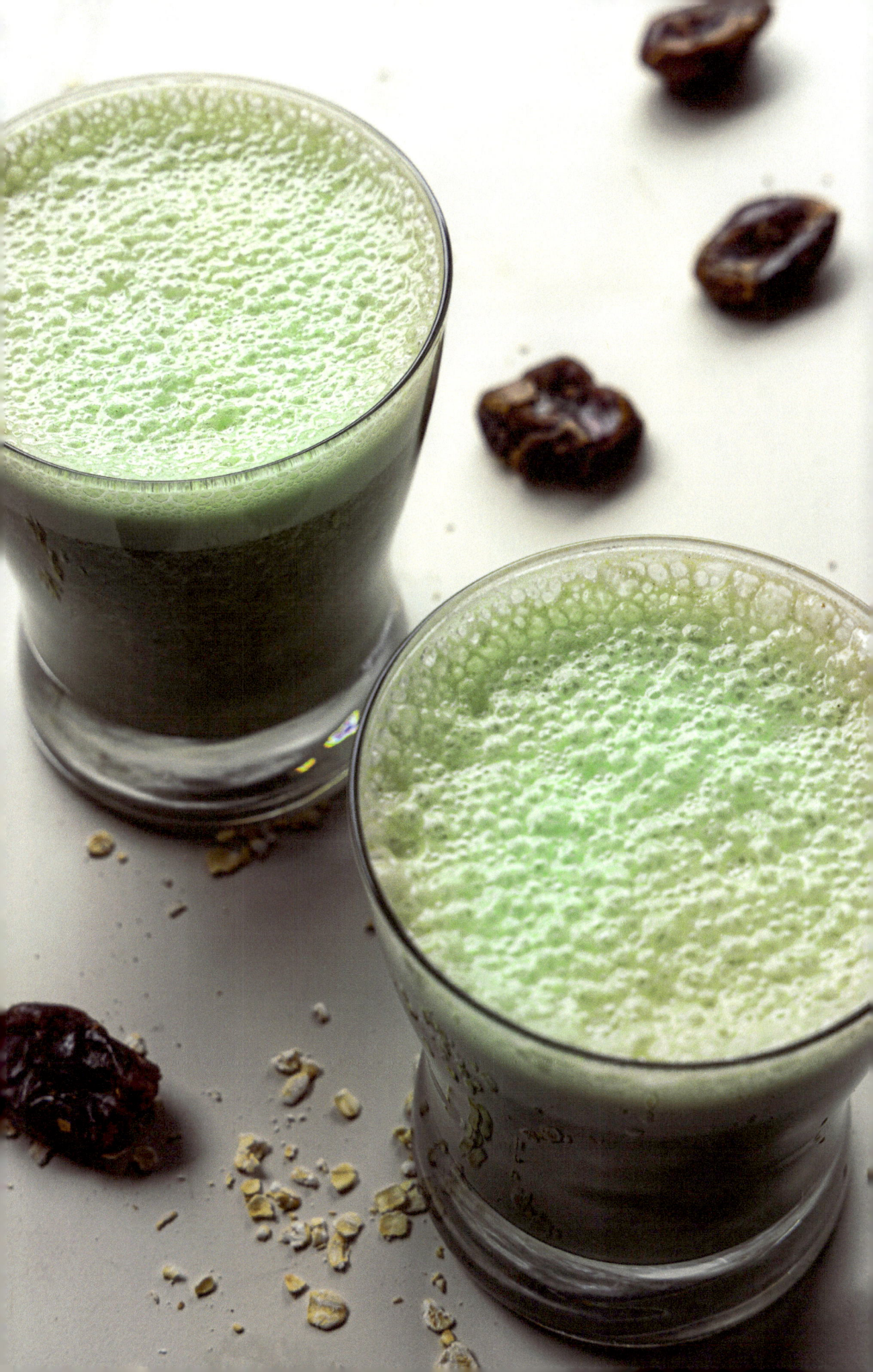

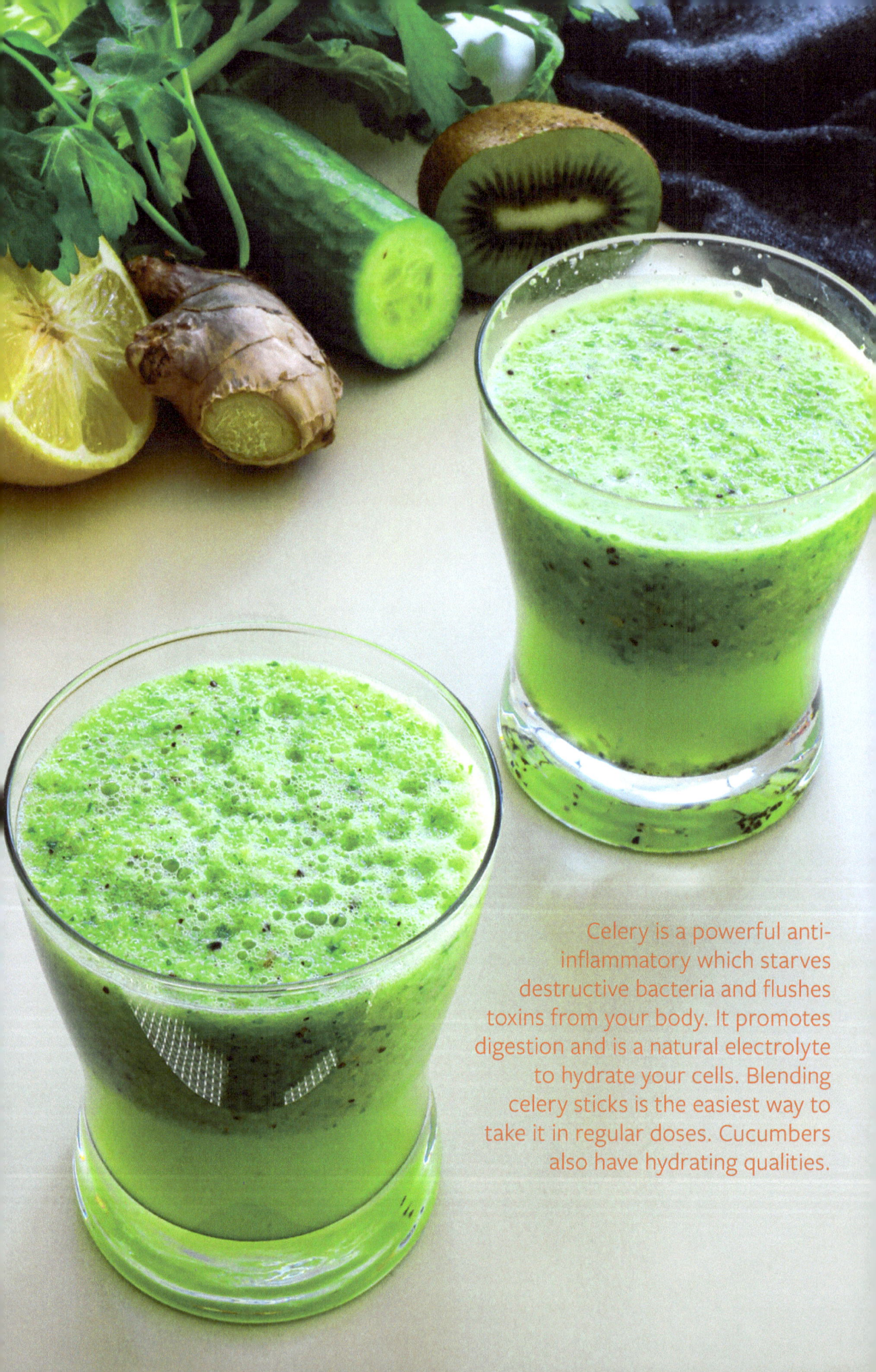

Celery is a powerful anti-inflammatory which starves destructive bacteria and flushes toxins from your body. It promotes digestion and is a natural electrolyte to hydrate your cells. Blending celery sticks is the easiest way to take it in regular doses. Cucumbers also have hydrating qualities.

GREEN JUICE

This juice is such an easy way to get nutrients and vitamins into your daily diet. I love making it as a substitute to a salad or cooked vegetables. It's quick to make and there's less to pack away. Your body's cells function better when slightly alkaline and green juices are perfect for achieving this. I make two juices while making dinner, one for that night and one for lunch the next day. Done!

PREP : 5 MINUTES | COOK : 0 MINUTES | SERVES : 1

1 cup chopped celery

1 kiwifruit, peeled

½ lemon, peeled

1cm piece of fresh ginger

½ cucumber

Small handful of parsley

Water

Add all the ingredients to your blender. Adjust your quantity of celery to suit your blender size.

Add water to the maximum level. Blend.

Ginger relaxes areas of tension like upset stomachs and helps to alleviate stress-related fatigue.

KIWIFRUIT IS THE ULTIMATE FRUIT FOR REGULATING BLOOD SUGAR LEVELS AND STRENGTHENING THE DIGESTIVE SYSTEM.

CALORIES 49KCAL | PROTEIN 2G | CARBS 9.8G | FATS 0.2G

ORANGE & APPLE JUICE

When I say "juice," I kind of mean "blend"... I use a NutriBullet which is actually a blender. There's nothing better, though, than getting the whole fruit in your drink. Remember that fruits are superfoods with anti-inflammatory properties that protect you from illness and disease. Citrus fruits should be a foundation in your diet. Apples play an important role in gut health and cleansing harmful bacteria and oranges protect our bodies from toxic heavy metals.

PREP : 5 MINUTES | COOK : 0 MINUTES | SERVES : 2

1 orange, peeled
1 apple, cored
½ lemon, peeled
Water

Cut your fruit in smaller pieces suitable for your blender.

Add about 500ml of cold water and blend.

THERE IS NO HARD AND FAST RULE FOR MIXING FRUITS IN DRINKS. ANYTHING WITH COLOUR IS LIFE-GIVING, SO FIND WAYS TO GET AS MANY FRUITS INTO YOUR DIET AS POSSIBLE.

CALORIES 59.5KCAL | PROTEIN 1.2G | CARBS 13G | FATS 0.3G

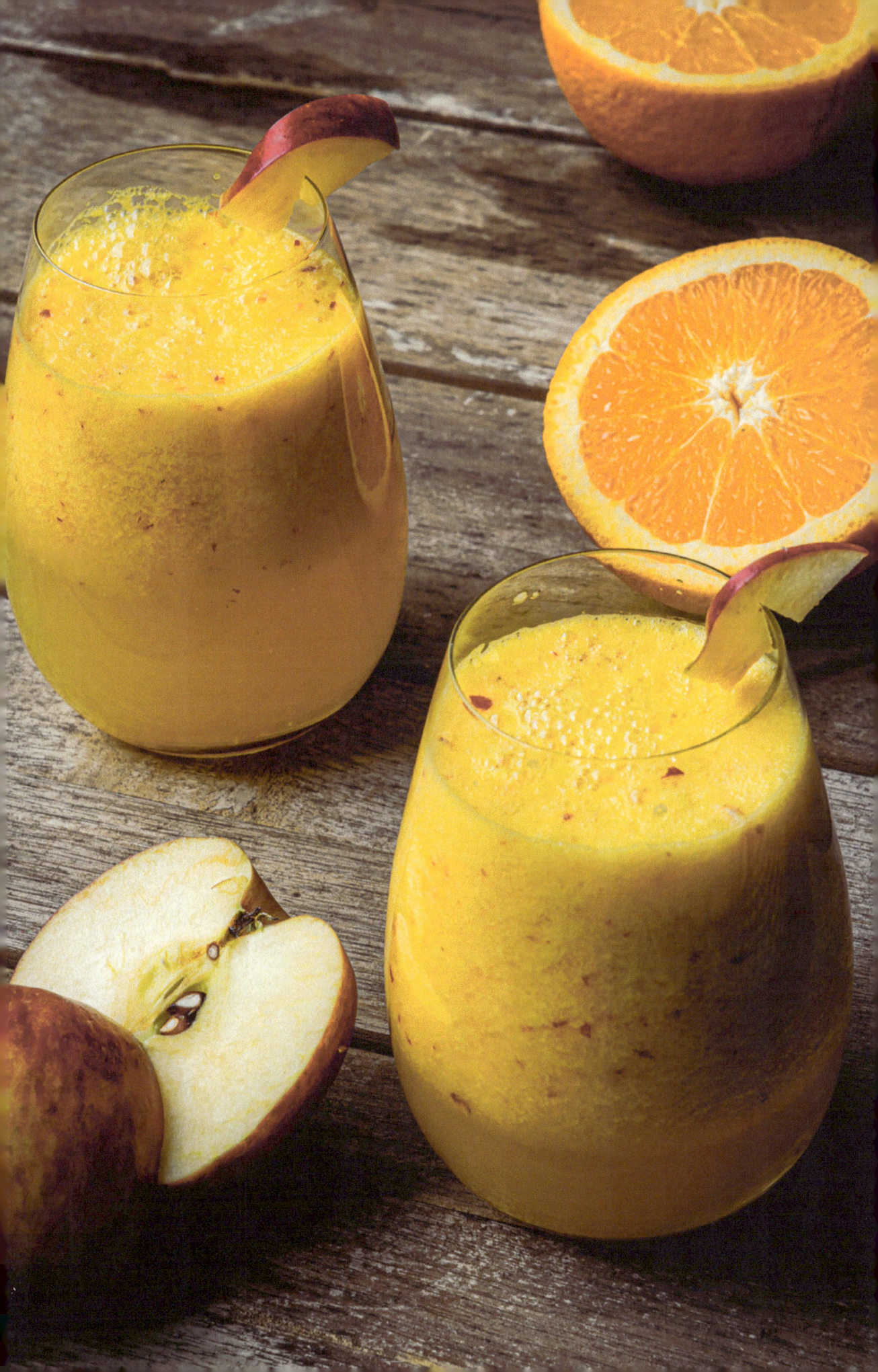

MACRONUTRIENT BREAKDOWN

PROTEINS - 4 calories per gram   CARBOHYDRATES – 4 calories per gram   FATS – 9 calories per gram

	FOOD	Serving Size (g)	Calories (kcal)	Protein (g)	Carbohydrates (g)	Fats (g)
PROTEINS	Chicken	200	207.2	44.6	0	3.2
	Beef	200	243.6	40.2	0	9.2
	Pork	200	221.6	48.2	0	3.2
	Salmon	200	400.7	41	0	26.3
	Ocean Trout	200	284.4	41.4	0	13.2
	Prawns	200	174.8	41	0	1.2
	Seafood Marinara	200	146.1	32.7	1.8	0.9
	Octopus	200	155.7	29.8	4.4	2.1
	Tuna in Olive Oil	200	447	44.4	3	28.6
	Turkey	200	232.2	43.2	0	6.6
	Turkey Patties	200	336.4	33	10.6	18
	Turkey Mince	200	244	33	1	12
	Kangaroo	200	212.8	39.6	4.6	4
	Eggs	6	436.5	39.6	0	30.9
	Yogurt	3 tbs (160g)	138	13.9	6.2	6.4
	Protein Powder	1 scoop (40g)	155.5	30	3.7	2.3
CARBOHYDRATES	Oats	1 cup	425.2	13.2	69.7	10.4
	White Rice	1 cup (185g cooked)	249.4	4.3	57.6	0.2
	Brown Rice	1 cup	236	4.6	50.8	1.6
	Couscous	1 cup	234.9	8	49.6	0.5
	Potato	1 cup (160g)	108.8	4.8	22.4	0
	Sweet potato	1 cup (160g)	155.6	4.6	34.3	0
	Pasta	1 cup	388	14.6	78.8	1.6
	Noodles	1 nest	201	5.6	42.4	1
	Bread (Sourdough Soy Lin)	2 slices	196.7	12.4	23.5	5.9
	Flour Tortillas	1 tortilla	123	4.1	18.1	3.8
FATS	Olive Oil	15ml (1 tbs)	123.3	0	0	13.7
	Coconut Oil	15ml (1 tbs)	81	0	0	9
	Peanut Oil	15ml (1 tbs)	124.2	0	0	13.8
	Peanut Butter	20ml (1 tbs)	119	5	2.7	9.8
	Avocado	260g (medium)	321.9	3.2	1	33.9
	Cashew Nuts	30g	173.6	5.1	5	14.8
	Pine Nuts	30g	209.8	3.9	1.3	21
	Almonds	30g	176.8	5.9	1.4	16.4
HERBS	Parsley	1 tsp (5g)	0	0	0	0
	Basil	1 tsp (5g)	0	0	0	0
	Oregano	1 tsp (5g)	0	0	0	0
	Mint	1 tsp (5g)	0	0	0	0
	Dill	1 tsp (5g)	0	0	0	0
	Thyme	1 tsp (5g)	0	0	0	0
	Rosemary	1 tsp (5g)	0	0	0	0
SPICES	Cinnamon	1 tsp (5g)	5.2	0	1.3	0
	Paprika	1 tsp (5g)	11.2	0	2.8	0
	Chilli Flakes	1 tsp (5g)	0	0	0	0
FRUIT	Apples	1 small	52.4	0.3	11.9	0.4
	Kiwi	1 medium	32.6	0.9	6.8	0.2
	Oranges	1 medium	60.2	1.6	13	0.2
	Bananas	1 medium	95.7	1.9	21.8	0.1
	Passionfruit	1 medium	11.6	1	1.9	0

	FOOD	Serving Size (g)	Calories (kcal)	Protein (g)	Carbohydrates (g)	Fats (g)
FRUIT	Blueberries	½ cup (50g)	36	0.5	8.5	0
	Raspberries	½ cup (50g)	17.2	0.6	3.7	0
	Strawberries	½ cup (50g)	8	0	2	0
	Lemon	1 medium	9.6	0.6	1.8	0
	Lime	1 small	4	0.4	0.6	0
	Dates	5 (30g)	97.2	0.6	23.7	0
	Pineapple	½ cup (50g)	16.4	0	4.1	0
	Watermelon	½ cup (50g)	12.8	0	3.2	0
	Frozen mixed berries	½ cup (50g)	16.8	0	4.2	0
VEGETABLES	Celery	1 cup	7.2	0.6	1.2	0
	Ginger	1 tsp (5g)	0	0	0	0
	Garlic	1 clove	0	0	0	0
	Mushrooms	1 cup	18	2.2	2.3	0
	Leafy Greens	1 cup	41.6	1.8	8.6	0
	Tomatoes	1 small (100g)	13.6	1	2.4	0
	Cucumber	1 small (100g)	8.8	0.4	1.8	0
	Broccoli	1 cup	31.2	7.2	0.6	0
	Corn	1 cup	96.4	4.6	15	2
	Green beans	1 cup (100g)	14.8	1.5	2.2	0
	Snow peas	1 cup (100g)	28.8	2.8	4.4	0
	Carrot	1 cup (100g)	25.6	0.9	5.5	0
	Shallots	1 tbs	0	0	0	0
	Chilli	1 small	10	0.6	1.9	0
	Olives	1 tbs (6)	165.6	0	0	18.4
	Capsicum	1 medium	30.7	2.1	4.9	0.3
	Beetroot	1 small (40g)	10.8	0.5	2.2	0
OTHER STAPLES	Honey	25g (1 tbs)	82	0	20.5	0
	Greek Coffee	1 tsp	17.6	0	4.4	0
	Milk	250ml	155.9	8.5	11.8	8.3
	Rice Packs	1 cup (120g)	188.1	5.1	37.2	2.1
	Salt & Pepper	1 tsp	0	0	0	0
	Flour	1 cup (155g)	536.7	16.7	113.2	1.9
	Bread crumbs	100g (⅔ cup)	370	14.2	68.4	4.4
	Bicarb Soda	1 tsp	0	0	0	0
	Greens superfood powder	1 tsp (4g)	8	0.6	1.4	0
	Psyllium husk	1 tbs (6g)	0.8	0.2	0	0
	Flaxseed meal	1 tbs (7g)	39.3	1.3	2	2.9
	Cocoa powder	1 tbs (8g)	23.6	1.3	1.9	1.2
	Dark chocolate 70% cocoa	4 squares (25g)	134.2	2.4	9.1	9.8
	Muesli	½ cup (60g)	238.7	5.6	35.4	8.3
	Chia seeds	1 tbs (15g)	62.9	3.1	0.7	5.3
	Passata	140g	33.5	2.1	5.6	0.3
	Crushed Tomatoes	1 can (410g)	72	4.4	13.6	0
	Sesame Oil	1 tsp (5g)	41.4	0	0	4.6
	Soy Sauce	1 tsp (5g)	8.8	0.8	1.4	0
	Bulgur	¼ cup (40g)	144.8	4.8	31.4	0
	Vanilla Extract	1 tbs (13g)	7.6	0	1.9	0
	Fetta Cheese	1 tbs (25g)	63.3	3.6	0.3	5.3
	Chicken Stock	1 cup (250ml)	28.6	5.9	0.8	0.2

MACRONUTRIENT BREAKDOWN

PROTEINS - 4 calories per gram   CARBOHYDRATES – 4 calories per gram   FATS – 9 calories per gram

	MEALS	Serving Size (g)	Calories (kcal)	Protein (g)	Carbohydrates (g)	Fats (g)
BREAKFASTS	Oats, Protein & Berries	1 cup	698.7	43.7	102.4	12.7
	Peanut Butter, Honey & Cinnamon on Toast	2 slices	516.7	22.4	49.4	25.5
	Scrambled Eggs & Avocado on Toast	2 slices	879.1	49.4	28.4	63.1
	Banana & Protein Pancakes	5 eggs	660.4	38.5	46.5	35.6
	Fluffy Banana Pancakes	2 pancakes	572.6	25.3	57.1	27
	Protein French Toast	2 slices	478.8	34.4	42.1	19.2
	Breakfast Burrito	2 wraps	745.5	36	39	49.5
	Greek coffee	1 cup	28.4	1.2	5.9	0
MEALS	Spaghetti Bolognese	200g	679.9	50.6	88.1	13.9
	Chargrilled Steak	300g	493.5	60.6	0.9	27.5
	Steak Sandwich	1 sandwich	565.8	41.5	30.2	31
	Meatballs / Meat Patties	180g	456.1	41.9	37.7	15.3
	Roasted Chicken Breast	250g	324.9	56	0.7	10.9
	Chicken Stir Fry	200g	340.4	47.9	12.9	10.8
	Chicken Schnitzel	200g	645.7	51.1	58.8	22.9
	Roasted Pork Loin	225g	314.1	54.4	0.5	10.5
	Chilli & Garlic Pasta	1 cup	640.2	15	79.8	29
	Fried Rice	1 cup	569.7	34.6	59.9	21.3
	Spaghetti Marinara	250g	743.4	56	82.6	21
	Ocean Trout & Prawns	300g	488.5	62.6	11.6	21.3
	Honey & Sesame Seed Salmon	200g	517.7	41.6	14.7	32.5
	Grilled Octopus	200g	233.1	30	5.1	10.3
	Chicken & Prawn Long Soup	300g	611.2	77.8	45.3	13.2
SIDES	Baked Potatoes (mix white/sweet)	2 cups (320g)	471.4	11	62.3	19.8
	Boiled Rice	1 cup (185g cooked)	249.4	4.3	57.6	0.2
	Chimichurri & Marinades	2 tbs	109.3	0.2	11.6	6.9
	Guacamole	3 tbs (160g)	188	2.1	1.7	19.2
	Steamed Vegetables	200g	45.2	5.2	5.2	0.4
	Tomato Pasta Sauce	½ cup (140g)	147.3	1.5	4.5	13.7
	Pesto Sauce	100g	179.2	1.1	0.5	19.2
	Greek salad	2 cups	212.2	0.8	2.3	22.2
	Tabouli	2 cups	437	7.8	39.8	27.4
	Bruschetta	1 slice	248.3	7.5	13.4	18.3
	Leafy Green Salad	1 cup	228.1	7.1	20	13.3
SNACKS	Yogurt, Protein, Berries & Muesli	3 tbs	478.5	39.5	43.9	16.1
	Ross Edgely Chocolate & Peanut Butter Cups	2 cups	120.8	2.7	5	10
SMOOTHIES & JUICES	Banana Protein Smoothie	1 shake	710.9	49.4	80.4	21.3
	Berries Protein Smoothie	1 shake	493.5	35.4	54	15.1
	Dates & Greens Protein Smoothie	1 shake	561	42.4	74.9	10.2
	Green Juice	1 drink	49	2	9.8	0.2
	Orange & Apple Juice	1 drink	59.5	1.2	13	0.3

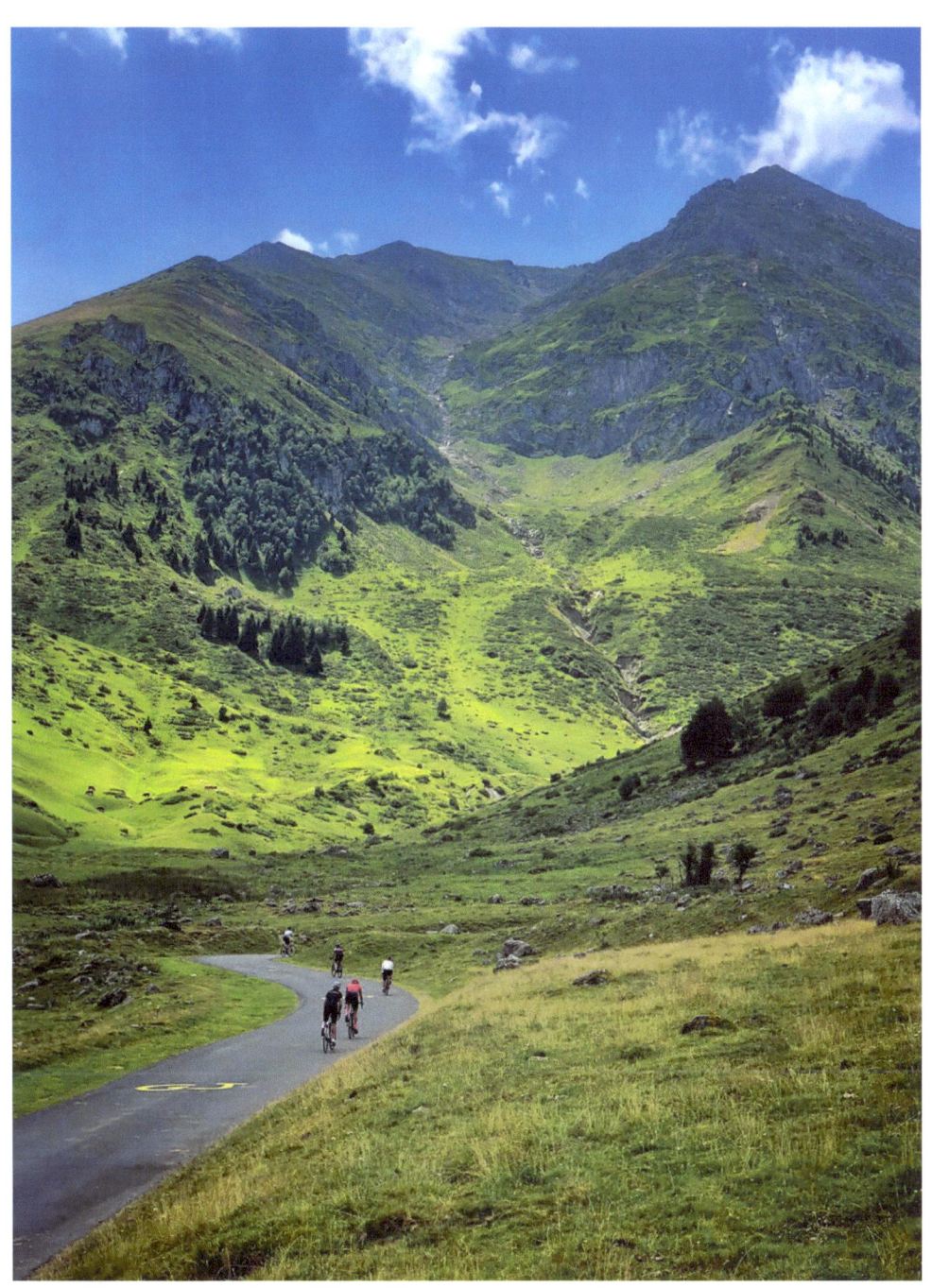

REFERENCES

BOOKS & ONLINE

Bulsiewicz, Dr. Will. *Fibre Fuelled: The Plant-Based Gut Health Plan to Lose Weight, Restore Health and Optimise Your Microbiome*. London, Penguin, 2022.

CalorieKing Australia. "Food Nutrition Facts and Free Calorie Counter." 2019. www.calorieking.com/au/en/.

Cavaliere, Jeff. ATHLEAN-XTM YouTube channel. www.youtube.com/c/athleanx/videos.

Edgley, Ross. *The Art of Resilience: Strategies for an Unbreakable Mind and Body*. London, HarperCollins Publishers, 2020.

Edgley, Ross. *Blueprint: Build a Bulletproof Body for Extreme Adventure in 365 days*. London, Dublin HarperCollins Publishers, 2021.

Edgley, Ross. *The World's Fittest Cookbook*. London, HarperCollins Publishers, 2022.

Edgley, Ross. YouTube channel. https://www.youtube.com/c/RossEdgley.

Fitzgerald, Matt. *Diet Cults: The Surprising Fallacy at the Core of Nutrition Fads and a Guide to Healthy Eating for the Rest of Us*. New York, Pegasus Books, 2014.

Gillespie, David. *Sweet Poison: Why Sugar Makes Us Fat*. Melbourne, Vic.: Penguin Random House, 2017.

Hay, Donna. *Off the Shelf: Cooking from the Pantry*. London, Fourth Estate, 2001.

Healthline. "Is Olive Oil a Good Cooking Oil? A Critical Look." 2018. www.healthline.com/nutrition/is-olive-oil-good-for-cooking#bottom-line.

Heart Foundation, The. "Fruit, Vegetables and Heart Health." www.heartfoundation.org.au/bundles/healthy-living-and-eating/fruit-vegetables-and-heart-health.

Hines, Luke. *Eat Clean & Feel Great with 100 Recipes for Real Food You Will Love!*. Sydney, Pan Macmillan Australia, 2016.

Holmes, Lee. *Supercharged: Eat Yourself Beautiful*. Sydney, Murdoch Books, 2014.

Manheim, Jason. *Superfood Juices, Smoothies & Drinks*. Sydney, Murdoch Books, 2016.

Marinos, S. "Foods to reduce stress: Fruit and vegetables linked to boosting mood." 2021. The House of Wellness. www.houseofwellness.com.au/health/nutrition/best-fruits-veggies-easing-stress.

MasterClass. *Learn the Differences Between a Saucepan and a Pot*. 2022. www.masterclass.com/articles/saucepan-vs-pot-explained#saucepan-vs-pot-what-are-the-main-differences.

Official Egg Info. "Egg White Vs Egg Yolk." www.egginfo.co.uk/egg-nutrition-and-health/egg-nutrition-information/white-and-yolk/compare#:~:text=Fats.

O'Hearn, Mike. YouTube channel. www.youtube.com/channel/UC8YnxGgVT62DDZ6sX1pLKGQ/videos.

Plitt, Greg. YouTube channel. www.youtube.com/channel/UCU6WaCIOCL_eToBcsBYFwAQ.

Ragusea, Adam. "Sharpening with a Whetstone: How to Get Started." www.youtube.com/watch?v=KY8jvFqpZ_o&t=1009s.

Ramsay, Gordon. YouTube channel. www.youtube.com/user/gordonramsay/.

William, Anthony. *Medical Medium. Life-Changing Foods: Save Yourself and the Ones You Love with the Hidden Healing Powers of Fruits and Vegetables*. Carlsbad, California: Hay House, Inc., 2016.

www.ingramcontent.com/pod-product-compliance
Lightning Source LLC
Chambersburg PA
CBHW041427010526
44107CB00045B/1525